Diabetes
Meal
Planner

Phil Vickery

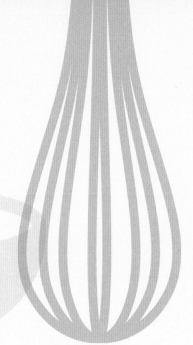

Diabetes Meal Planner

DELICIOUSLY SIMPLE RECIPES AND WEEKLY WEIGHT-LOSS MENUS

Phil Vickery

with Bea Harling BSc

K

All nutritional analyses are calculated per portion.

An Hachette UK Company
www.hachette.co.uk

First published in Great Britain in 2020 by
Kyle Books, an imprint of Kyle Cathie Ltd
Carmelite House
50 Victoria Embankment
London EC4Y 0DZ
www.kylebooks.co.uk

ISBN: 978 0 85783 778 3

The publisher will donate 2% of the recommended retail price of every
book purchased in the UK to Diabetes UK (except where sold at more than
52.4% discount to the RRP, where the donation will be 1.2–1.6%)

Editorial Director: Judith Hannam
Project Editor: Claire Rogers
Editorial Assistant: Florence Filose
Design: Paul Palmer-Edwards
Photography: Kate Whitaker
Food styling: Annie Rigg
Production: Katherine Hockley

A Cataloguing in Publication record for this title is available from
the British Library.

Printed and bound in China

10 9 8 7 6 5 4 3 2 1

Contents

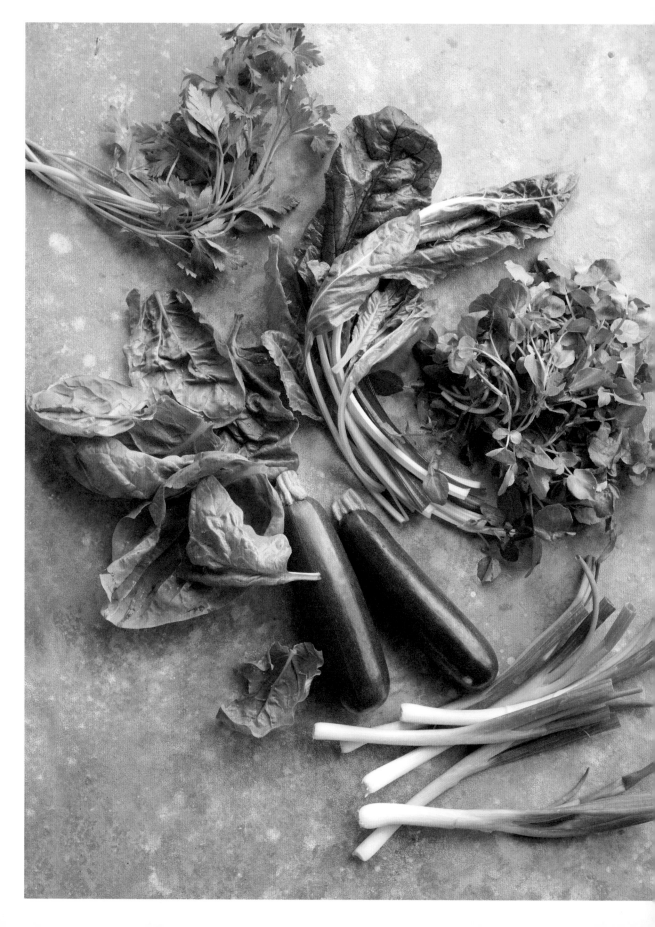

Foreword

Hello,

Thank you for buying this book.

Diabetes is with you when you go to sleep. It's with you when you wake up. It's also with you every mealtime, and it's far from simple.

But planning what you eat and having some go-to recipes that you know are good for you can make life with diabetes easier.

This book will help you plan, make and eat delicious, healthier meals. By buying it you're supporting our vital work.

Whether it's through our helpline, local groups or website, you'll be helping us provide the information and support that people need to live well with diabetes.

Our campaigns change thousands of people's lives every year and ensure care is always getting better. Our researchers are discovering more about diabetes, helping us find new treatments and reducing the damage it does every day. We're fighting for a world where diabetes can do no harm. You can join us at www.diabetes.org.uk.

Thank you for your support, and enjoy the book.

Best wishes,

Chris Askew
Chief Executive, Diabetes UK

Introduction

When Bea Harling and I set out to write our first diabetes book, *The Ultimate Diabetes Cookbook*, in 2016, we really had no idea how the book would be received. As with many of the books I have written, I thought it would be a relatively straightforward case of developing and cooking the recipes, getting them photographed and saying, 'hey ho, that's it'. We soon realised it wouldn't be as simple as that.

The list of ingredients that you can eat if you have diabetes is fortunately very varied, but when you are building balanced, nutritional recipes, you really need to be extremely careful, and it takes a huge amount of time and effort to get things right. As with any very focused recipe development, you have to be so strict, not only when developing or cooking the recipes, but also to ensure you give the correct advice. Research is being published all the time and there have been significant changes even in the three years since the publication of *The Ultimate Diabetes Cookbook*.

We have tried to write easy, colourful and tasty recipes that hopefully will inspire you to get involved and cook. In addition, we've given you sample low-calorie menus, using these recipes, for those wanting to lose weight to help manage their diabetes, to help you plan every meal of the day for two weeks. We have also taken into consideration shopping and so have kept ingredients to a minimum. Some recipes are very simple, and we make no excuse for that – as a wise chef once said to me, 'The fewer ingredients, the less you can hide.'

Always, the overriding factor is the need to eat a nutritionally well-balanced diet, keeping a careful eye on calorie intake if you're trying to manage your weight, but also it goes without saying that keeping active is crucial. As you know, I am no doctor, but my older brother is, so we often chat about diets, and he always stresses the need for a combination of moderate exercise and a balanced diet.

Every word in this book has been checked by Diabetes UK and they have been invaluable with guidance, help and latest research. Please note, though, that before embarking on any diet, you should seek advice from your doctor or healthcare professional.

Phil Vickery

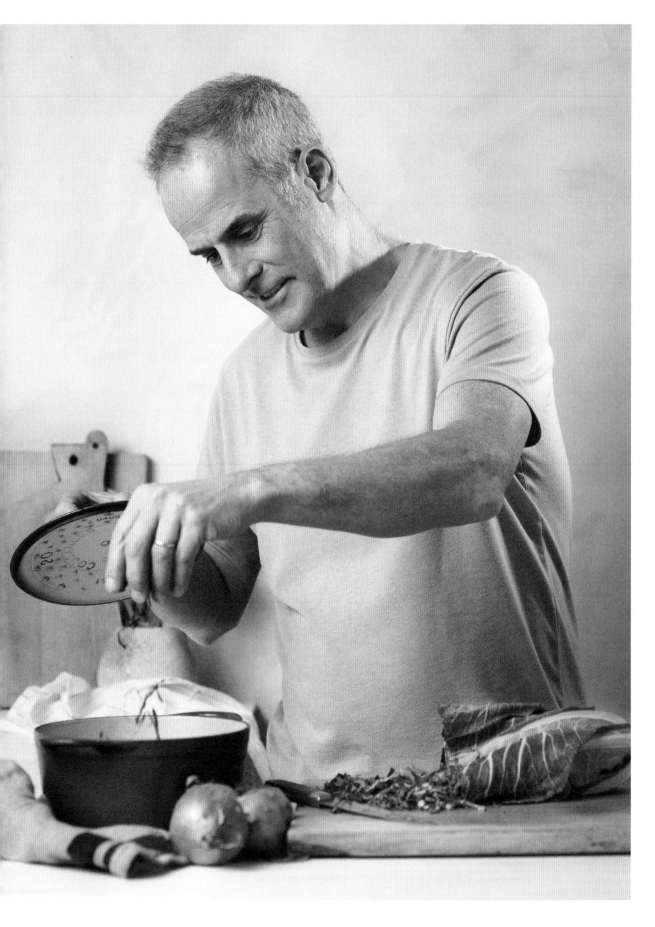

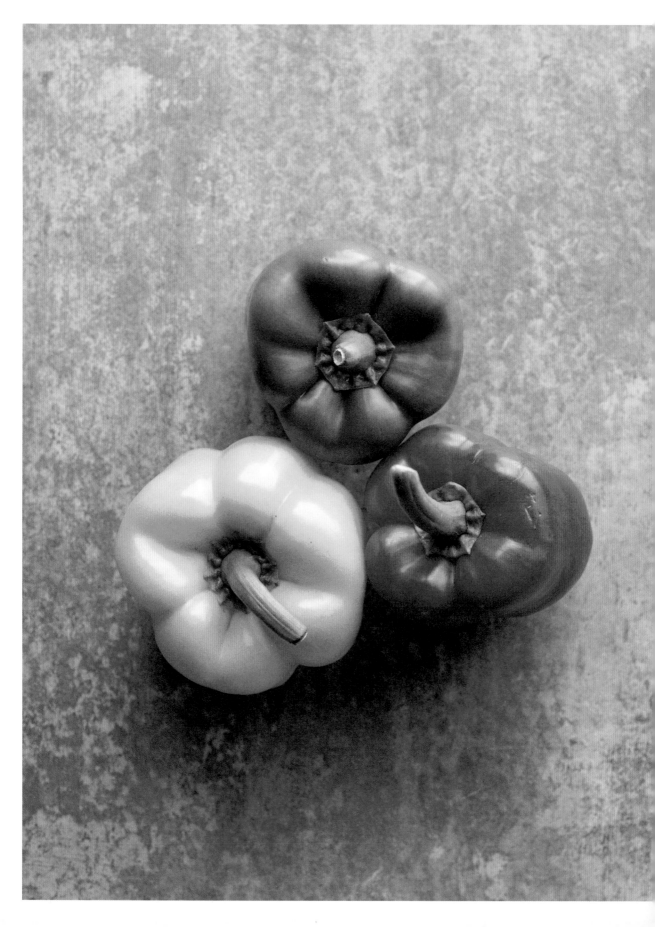

What is diabetes?

More people than ever have diabetes – it affects more people than all cancers and dementia combined. It is not always the easiest of conditions to understand and not enough people appreciate the damage it can do. Symptoms include being unusually thirsty, feeling tired all the time and needing to pee more than usual. By spotting the symptoms early, taking prescribed medications and making healthy changes to diet and lifestyle, you can reduce your chances of developing diabetes complications.

Diabetes is a condition where someone has too much glucose (sugar) in their blood. When people don't have diabetes, their blood sugar levels are controlled by a hormone, insulin, which is produced in their pancreas. Insulin helps to move glucose from our blood into our cells, such as muscles, where it is used as fuel for energy.

There are two main types of diabetes – type 1 and type 2. Ninety percent of people with diabetes have the type 2 version; 8 per cent have type 1, and about 2 per cent of people have rarer types of diabetes. Rarer forms of diabetes include monogenic diabetes, cystic fibrosis-related diabetes and diabetes caused by rare syndromes. Certain types of medication, such as steroids and antipsychotics, surgery or hormonal imbalances can also lead to other types of diabetes.

Type 1 develops when the insulin-producing cells in the body have been destroyed and the body is unable to produce any insulin. It can develop at any age but usually appears before the age of 40, and especially in childhood. It is not caused by diet or lifestyle – a common misconception. We don't know the exact cause, so there is currently no cure and the long-term health risks are serious: everyone with type 1 needs to treat their diabetes by injecting insulin or using an insulin pump, as well as eating healthily and being regularly active.

Type 2 develops when the body either can't produce enough insulin to keep blood glucose levels in check, or can't use insulin properly. As a result, glucose is poorly absorbed, and the excess can be stored as fat: often around the tummy and clogging up the liver and pancreas. Longer-term health risks are serious. It usually strikes in midlife and slightly more men than women are affected by type 2 diabetes. The risk increases as you get older, although in people of South Asian descent, who are at greater risk overall, the chances increase from the age of 25. People from African-Caribbean and Black African backgrounds are also at higher risk of developing it. Having a close family member with diabetes (a sibling or parent) and being overweight also increases your risk.

Becoming more active

The NHS website is a great resource for inspiration, free exercise programmes (without equipment) and tips on staying healthy and living well: have a browse. If you don't do much activity, it's best to start slowly and gradually build up, and check with your doctor.

Over a week, aim to do around two and a half hours of moderate activities that leave you mildly out of breath; such as walking, easy cycling or swimming. Ideally mix aerobic fitness like this with exercises that improve muscle strength, on at least two days a week.

Why a healthy, balanced diet is important

People with diabetes spend around three hours with a healthcare professional every year; for the remaining 8,757 hours they must manage their diabetes themselves. An important part of this self-care is eating a healthy, balanced diet. There isn't a special diet for people with diabetes; dietary guidelines are very similar to those recommended for everyone. Making healthier food choices is good for everybody.

This means including more of certain foods: whole grains, fruit, plenty of vegetables, especially green leafy varieties and pulses like beans and lentils. Incorporate healthy fats: oily fish, for example, avocado and nuts. Eat less of other types of food such as: highly refined grains and processed meats. Reduce added sugar, sugary food and drinks. Lower salt and saturated fat. Eat less red meat, maybe once or twice a week only and choose better quality, if possible.

Before making any changes to your diet, it is best to check with your healthcare team first, especially if the diet is restrictive and/or you're on diabetes medication. Unless advised by your team, it's best to eat a variety of healthy foods rather than take vitamin and mineral supplements, to get the essential nutrients and manage your diabetes.

- **Don't bother with so-called 'diabetic food', it has no special benefit.**

- Make some of your exercise social: get the support of other people, friends and family. Join a group or an online community to make it a more enjoyable experience. Sharing the journey, and maybe having some fun, will help you to stay motivated along the way.

- Begin by setting a small and realistic goal. Listen to music during a simple workout.

- Vary the walk, class or type of exercise regularly, to learn something new.

- Pre-book exercise classes for the week: this can help establish them as part of your routine.

You can help manage your diabetes by:

- Following a healthy, balanced diet.

- Losing weight if you are overweight. Maintaining a healthy weight will enable your body to use insulin better and reduces the risk of long-term diabetes complications.

- Drinking alcohol sensibly, if you drink. Keeping everything in moderation is a good rule of thumb, especially around alcohol.

- Stopping smoking.

- Taking regular exercise. Look at diet and exercise together. Anything is better than nothing (and more is better).

Ten Top Tips

1. Choose healthier carbohydrates

All carbohydrates (starch, sugar and fibre) affect blood sugar levels, so you need to keep an eye on the amount you eat. What's most important is the type of carbohydrate you choose. Carbohydrates are an important source of energy, so it's not good to exclude them. There is some confusion surrounding carbs and not everyone agrees on the same approach. Sensibly, choosing healthier carbs and reducing your intake of the rest is better for your health.

Minimally processed whole grains such as brown rice or pasta, oats and buckwheat are healthy sources of carbohydrate that release energy more slowly, keeping you feeling full, and provide vitamins, minerals, fibre and a host of phytonutrients. The presence of fibre, fat and protein in food slows down the absorption and digestion of carbs and produces a smaller rise in blood sugar. Wholewheat pasta in particular has a far lower glycaemic response than white pasta, meaning it has a smaller effect on blood glucose levels.

Unhealthier sources of carbs include highly processed foods, which are much lower in nutritional quality and tend to raise your blood sugar more rapidly, which can be problematic for managing diabetes. Cut down on refined grains like white rice and foods like cakes, pastries and white bread. Legumes, which include pulses, chickpeas, beans and lentils, are an inexpensive source of healthy carbohydrates, protein, vitamins and fibre. Other healthy sources of carbohydrates include unsweetened yogurt (dairy), fruit and veg.

2. Eat more fruit and veg

Variety is as important as quantity and the advice to make a colourful plate of veg and fruit still holds good. Antioxidants, polyphenols and phytonutrients are natural protectors in plants that also benefit us when we eat them. Some are concentrated in the skin pigments, so leave the peel on if you can (and for valuable fibre). Fresh fruit and vegetables, and the fibre they contain, also work to keep hunger pangs under control.

Eat your five a day: a portion is about 80g, or roughly a handful. Fresh, frozen, dried and canned all count towards your total. Don't forget to include the vegetables you add when cooking, like onions, or tomatoes in a pasta sauce. Potatoes don't count because they mainly contribute starch, so fall into the starchy carbohydrate food group. Eating a variety of non-starchy veg and fruit each day gives your body the mix of beneficial nutrients it needs.

You may ask, 'Can I eat fruit if I have diabetes?'. Yes. Although we know fruits and vegetables are good for us, people with diabetes are often told they can't eat fruit because it is too sweet or contains sugar. Whole fruit is good for everyone. It contains natural sugar. Fruit juice and smoothies mostly have the fibre squeezed out and so it becomes 'free' sugar. Restrict these to one small 150ml glass a day.

Some fruits such as tropical fruit (mangoes, for example) are higher in sugar than other fruits like apples and berries. So the practical answer is to have smaller portions.

Snack on raw vegetables: make vegetables more interesting: stir-fry or steam, then add a pinch of spice and herbs. Take a fresh look at soups; they are cheap and practical.

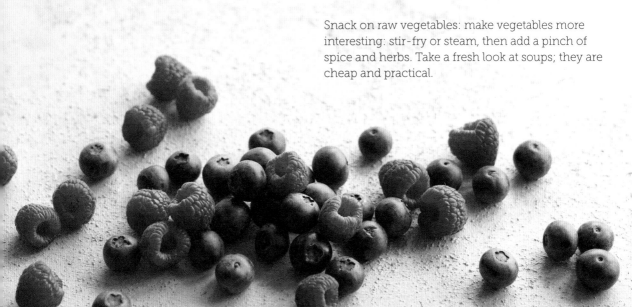

3. Choose fibre

Fibre comes in two varieties, both of which are beneficial to health: insoluble and soluble fibre. Good sources of fibre are whole grains, oat and wheat bran, fresh fruits and vegetables, legumes and nuts. Fibre-rich foods keep you feeling full and help to control the release of sugar into your blood, because they slow digestion. Fibre also plays an important part in gut health, feeding the flora of bacteria we need for good health.

- Eat whole fruits instead of a fruit juice drink.

- Choose rice, cereals, bread and pasta with wholegrain products over white.

- Swap beans or legumes for meat, a few times a week in meals.

- Increase the amount of fibre you eat gradually rather than suddenly.

- Drink more water and fluids when you make healthy changes and increase fibre intake, because it absorbs water.

4. Eat less salt

A surprising amount of salt in our daily diet comes from processed and prepared foods, like packaged snacks, breakfast cereal, bread and restaurant meals. It's worth keeping an eye on the product labels: keep in mind a maximum of 6 grams or one teaspoon of salt a day.

- Cut back on prepared, processed foods and replace with more fresh ingredients. You are then in control of the ingredients in your meals and this will also give you the chance to reduce your intake of salt.

- Eat smaller portions of salty foods.

- Experiment with more herbs and spices, instead of salt. Citrus like lemon activates similar taste sensors to sodium and can provide more flavour with less salt.

Leave the pepper pot on the table and put the salt back in the cupboard. One of the easiest ways to cut down on salt is to use herbs and spices, both dried and fresh. Think garlic, ginger, citrus, vinegar, cinnamon, turmeric, basil, chilli and combinations like dukkha (roasted nuts and spices), inspired by food in the Middle East. Ideas for more flavours to make meals and vegetable sides more interesting can be borrowed from world cuisine: healthy ideas, exciting new flavours.

Focus on enhancing natural flavour: ingredients with strong flavours, like dried mushrooms, are great replacements for salt. Add a pinch of spice (nutmeg is a natural) to steamed greens or scrambled eggs.

Umami or, put simply, 'savouriness' is detected by one of our taste senses. Cooking with foods naturally high in L-glutamate (which triggers our umami taste receptors), such as mushrooms, tomatoes, seaweed, carrots and Chinese cabbage, adds a delicious depth of flavour. Do note, though, that soy sauce, fish sauce, miso and mature cheeses are high in umami but also in salt.

5. Include a variety of proteins

Don't worry too much about the amount of protein to eat; it's more important to include a variety of healthy proteins. Choose chicken, turkey, beans, eggs, salmon (people with diabetes should have two portions of oily fish per week), tofu and whole grains over less healthy options of red and processed meats. Try 'meatless Mondays' to include plant-based proteins: pulses, beans, nuts and seeds. Protein-rich foods like fish and eggs can be the simplest fast food, quick to cook and, combined with whole grains, ensure a good supply of the amino acids you need.

6. Know your fats

Eating healthier types of fat is better for your cholesterol levels and heart health. Reducing overall fat intake is still important if you need to lose weight; fat is fat and – however it is packaged – it is high in calories. But low-fat and no-fat foods are not always the best way to go: some fats can be beneficial (see below), and much of the pre-packaged food labelled as 'low fat' can contain extra added sugar. Instead it is the type of fat that is important.

Fats to avoid are trans and partially hydrogenated fat found in processed food like spreads, pastries and biscuits. Aim to cut down on eating foods high in saturated fats, such as in animal products and red meat. You can check saturated fats on food labels:

- High: More than 5g saturates per 100g. May be labelled with red.

- Medium: 1.5–5g saturates per 100g. Usually amber.

- Low: less than 1.5g saturates per 100g. Usually green.

To control the amount of fat you use for frying, baking and roasting, you can get a handy little spray bottle containing vegetable oil. One spray is equivalent to 1 calorie and goes further, so you can cut down on the amount of oil needed.

Embrace healthy fat, found in plant foods, nuts and seeds, and unsaturated fats in vegetable and olive oils, avocado and dairy products. For those who are not vegetarian, oily fish like salmon, mackerel and trout are full of good fats. Oily fish also provides omega-3, which can help protect the heart. Aim to have 2 portions of oily fish a week.

Do include some dairy foods every day, like yogurt and milk. Dairy products are good sources of protein, some vitamins and calcium. Evidence shows us that the type of saturated fat found in dairy may actually be beneficial to our heart health. Try to choose unsweetened versions. You could try swapping some of the low-fat dairy in the recipes for some whole fat unsweetened dairy. Some studies suggest that healthy fats may slow the release of sugars from starchy carbs. Plus, fat is a slow-burn source of energy and it doesn't encourage insulin spikes.

Of course, you do need to be mindful of foods high in fat, because they are also naturally high in calories. That said, some types of fat are actually good for us and have nutritional benefits. While the message about 'low-fat' foods has created some fear surrounding any food high in fat, it is good to know that nuts and seeds contain the good, beneficial, healthy fat. Restrict the amount to a small handful.

7. Cut down on added sugar

Sugars can be natural, such as those found in dairy foods (lactose) and in vegetables and fruit (fructose). Then there are the added, or 'free', sugars that you add yourself or are added by the manufacturer in foods such as sweets, chocolate and sugary drinks. Free sugars also include the natural sugars in maple syrup, honey and agave, as well as the sugar in juices and smoothies – all of these foods also need to be limited in your diet. Without the fibre of the whole food, the sugar is quickly digested and not satisfying for long. The problem is, you could drink several hundred calories in a glass much faster than you could chew and digest the equivalent whole fruit. Whole fruits contain natural sugar and many other beneficial nutrients, so are the best choice.

Retrain your taste buds. You can learn to enjoy foods with less sugar – honest! The same goes with salt. Make the change and reduce the amount gradually and consistently over a period of time. Try low sugar rather than none: that is much harder to start with. Do it slowly over time and you are much more likely to succeed in making it a permanent habit. The messages from your brain will retreat, and your taste for other flavours will kick in.

To help you make a start, you could also try an artificial sweetener. For more information, read the section on sugar, sweeteners and diabetes at www.diabetes.org.uk.

8. Be smart with snacks

Avoiding snacks is the best policy and, even smarter, try to keep yourself feeling full instead: try making a hot drink when you feel like reaching for a snack. If you snack, choose whole fruit, cherry tomatoes, pepper strips, carrot sticks and unsweetened yogurts.

A few unsalted, unflavoured nuts with 'good' fats can curb appetite: unsalted nuts and seeds are an all-round good snack. Be mindful that they are also high in calories, but an occasional handful as a snack is a good thing. Skin-on nuts are high in fibre and protein, and fill you up instead of sugary snacks. Mix the nuts with seeds and toast them on a tray in a hot oven for a few minutes, then keep them in a jar. Add spices for a savoury kick.

9. Drink plenty of water

There are many options for what to drink, but water is best. Regardless, it's important to drink enough fluid. A general guide is around eight to ten cups or glasses a day. especially when you are adding more fibre to your diet. Although all drinks count, go for water, unsweetened, or no-calorie and sugar-free drinks. Use a refillable water bottle and make your own infused drinks. Try pouring yourself a chilled, sparkling water with a splash of citrus juice or mint and cucumber. (Limit the amount of fruit juice, smoothies and sugary, fizzy drinks for calories' sake; they also rapidly affect your blood sugar levels.) Drink water flavoured with mint, sparkling or hot, infused with tea or ginger, or however you want, to make water more interesting for you.

10. Moderate your alcohol intake

If you do drink, spread it out over a week to avoid binges and make a few days each week alcohol free.

Creating good eating habits

Eating is a confusing business with so much conflicting information around. Decide what you are aiming for and just become more aware of what you are eating. Then take positive action from the suggestions in the Ten Top Tips above. To begin, just start slowly, making some simple changes to your diet, exercise and lifestyle.

Below are some tips that will also help you create good habits. Some of them may seem very obvious, but it's worth trying them out.

Plan in advance

Preparation is key to have tasty food ready to make at home or packed up for lunch. Write your shopping list before heading out shopping and ideally look ahead for the week. Having some satisfying, healthy options may make you less inclined to buy junk food.

Cook in bulk

Make your freezer your friend. Make double quantities when you can, eat some and freeze the rest in portions for the microwave.

Use frozen vegetables

These are a great way of getting your five a day: they need less prep time and are easy to cook (use a microwave or steam, rather than boiling). It's simple to control portion size and creates less waste from veg sitting in the fridge until spoiled, and they are often higher in nutrients as they are picked and frozen when very fresh. Best of all, they are available in your kitchen when you need something quick.

Key kitchen tip

Invest in a good-quality pan with a heavy base that transfers the heat well; it will cook food better and with less oil. Keep a pump bottle or spray oil next to the cooker.

Use simple cooking techniques

To preserve more nutrients in vegetables, concentrate flavours and use less oil and salt, all you need to do is grill, steam, sauté, sear and roast.

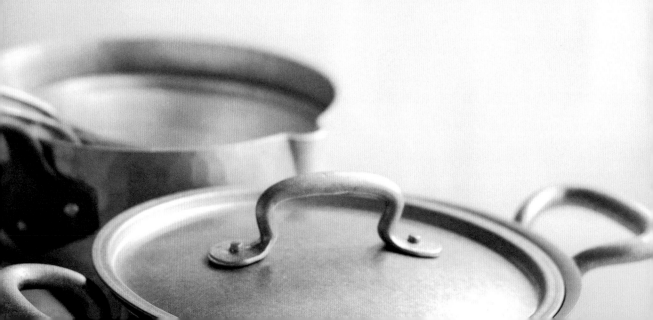

Use less meat
In recipes, try reducing the meat portion and stretch it out with extra vegetables, beans or pulses instead.

Eat slowly and use a small plate
This helps to fool yourself into eating a smaller portion. Portion out food and don't leave the serving dish on the table for seconds.

Out of sight out of mind
Reorganise your kitchen and put healthier foods like fruit in the first visible position. Clear out things like family sized 'share' packets of sweets and crisps or chocolate biscuits.

Sleep
Aim to get an early night and seven to eight hours sleep, when you can.

When the wheels fall off your plan...
Don't beat yourself up. It happens. Just (keep calm and) carry on.

Why less is better
To maintain a healthy weight, keep a keen eye on portion sizes. Simply eating a little less every day will keep you on the right track to a better weight. It's difficult to guess at a portion and to get it right. Remember, everybody's needs are different and your weight, gender, body composition and activity levels all make a difference. A dietitian will be able to advise you on the portion sizes that are right for you. Search www.diabetes.org.uk for a visual guide to portion sizes.

Weekly menu plans
At the back of the book are low-calorie menu plans for those who have been advised to lose weight to help manage their diabetes. See page 160.

Be a savvy shopper
Start looking at the labels on food packaging. 'Back-of-pack' labelling – found by law on both food and drink products – gives essential information about the ingredients, nutritional composition (calories, fats, sugars, salt, etc.) and known allergens. The ingredients are listed in order, starting with the highest-quantity ingredient first and ending the lowest-quantity ingredient last. If sugar appears in the first three, that food is likely to be high in sugar.

Colour-coded labelling
Colour-coded labelling – known as 'traffic light' labelling – is an easy way to check at a glance how healthy a food or drink is, based on how much fat, saturated fat, sugars and salt it contains. The amounts are colour-coded green to red to show whether a particular nutrient is low (green), medium (amber) or high (red). Always try to choose foods with more greens and few ambers. Only have reds occasionally and have smaller portions.

All the recipes in this book have traffic light labelling and nutritional analysis. The quantity (in grams) of the fat, sat fat, sugar and salt is given per portion below the colour-coded labels.

All the recipes that are vegan or gluten-free are also labelled as follows:

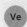 Vegan

 Gluten-free

Store-cupboard staples
Stock up on a few dried, canned and frozen stores so that you have ingredients on hand for making fresh, quick meals.

- Grains in their whole form, such as brown rice, rolled oats and cracked wholegrain wheat. These offer a complete package of health benefits from fibre, protein, vitamins and minerals.

- Pulses are the edible seeds from a legume plant. Examples include kidney and black beans, chickpeas and lentils. Pulses are an inexpensive source of protein, vitamins, healthy carbohydrates and fibre.

- Beans also have a useful number of polyphenols: the darker the bean, the more they contain. So, stir in some beans next time you are cooking rice, or a main meal. Try out a new variety of bean each week.

- See page 170 for more suggestions.

Dried pasta shapes made from bean or lentil flour
These are really worth a try instead of the usual refined wheat pasta; the flavour is good, and the change will boost a whole range of nutrients in one meal. Cooking pasta al dente makes it slower to digest as does chilling cooked pasta or processed rice and starchy carbs; even if you reheat it after, this helps to make the starch resistant to fast digestion. Follow food safety guidelines when cooling, storing and reheating foods in order to minimise the risk of potential food poisoning.

Follow this general method of preparing most dried whole grains and pulses before using in recipes, to make them digestible: Place them in a glass bowl with double the volume of cold water. Cover and leave overnight. Drain and rinse; they are now ready to cook. Keep in the fridge for up to 3 days.

It is best to check the pack instructions for cooking grains and pulses because the same ingredient can be processed differently: some need soaking and some are 'quick cook' for convenience. If the long cooking time puts you off, go for the canned versions of chickpeas, lentils, etc. You can find inspired combinations of whole grains, seeds and pulses in ready-to-heat pouches and they make wonderful shortcuts.

Buckwheat
A versatile fruit seed, related to rhubarb and sorrel, not wheat at all. It is a heart-healthy option because it contains rutin, a type of fibre that protects against the effects of high cholesterol. It's rich in magnesium (for healthy bones and muscle function) and zinc (good for your skin health), plus iron. The whole grains are a great base to use instead of all rice, for risottos and salads. Try swapping in some buckwheat flour in baking and breakfast pancakes. The flavour can taste bitter to some people; always rinse and try sparingly first. See the recipe on page 31.

Lentils
Although they include all the beneficial nutrients like fibre, protein, minerals and vitamins, lentils are low in calories. They are perfect to eat in warming casseroles in winter, in the summer added to salads, or puréed in spreads, for crudité and crackers. An easy way to add the useful nutrients from lentils is to purée them after cooking and use to thicken soups and sauces. See the recipes on pages 100, 102 and 134.

Amaranth
A small seed-like grain, rich in iron and a source of protein. Swap some into porridge, such as the recipe on page 31, for a great breakfast alternative.

Bulgar wheat
A form of whole wheat that has been parboiled and dried, making it a quicker to cook. You can find packs of quick-cook wholewheat bulgar mixed with other grains such millet and red rice: lovely in warm salads. Contains useful fibre as well as supplying energising B vitamins. Try serving with chilli (see page 103) or tagine (see page 107).

Quinoa
This grain-like seed contains more protein than most other grains. It is a good source of iron and calcium. To cook from dry, rinse the quinoa (to remove a slightly bitter coating on the seeds). Place it in a pan with half a reduced-salt stock cube, if you like, and cover it with the water. Bring to the boil and cook for 12–15 minutes (you will see the little 'tails' appear). Leave to cool and drain well. Spread it over a shallow dish to dry and fluff up. See the recipes on pages 64 and 92.

Oats
These make a good contribution of protein, calcium and essential fatty acids. Oats also contain a soluble fibre, beta-glucan, and eating them regularly can offer the benefit of helping to lower blood cholesterol levels. You can also find packets of oat bran (a by-product of making flour from whole oats); adding a spoonful of this in with the oats you are cooking is a good tip to boost the beta-glucan even more.

You will see many types available, processed in different ways, from jumbo to fine – and the size of the grain really does count. Jumbo rolled oats are better than quick-cook and instant oats as they are slower to digest than the more processed variety and cause less of a rise in blood sugar levels after eating. See the recipes on pages 31 and 32.

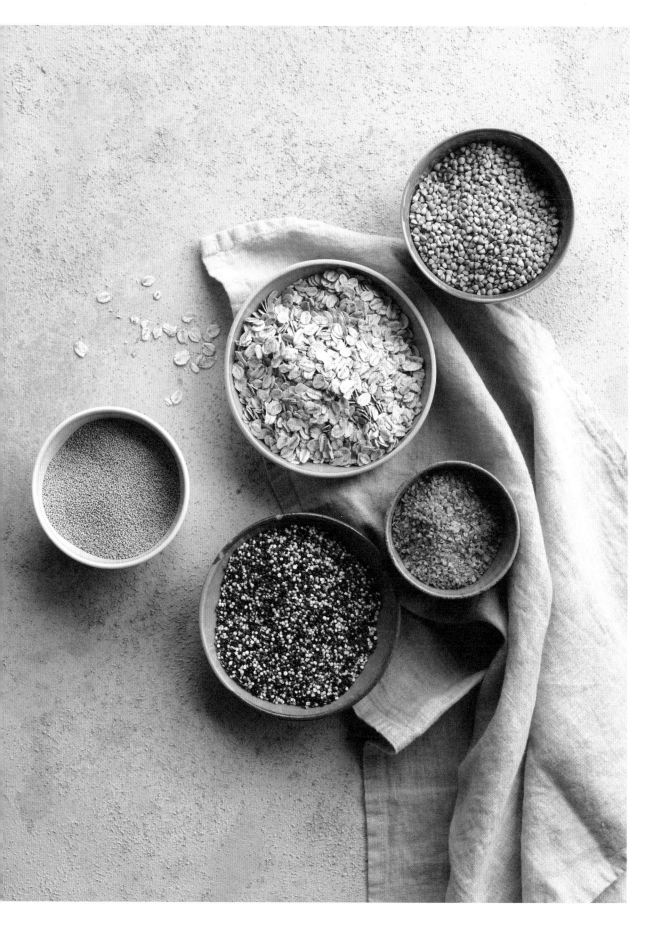

Balanced
Breakfast

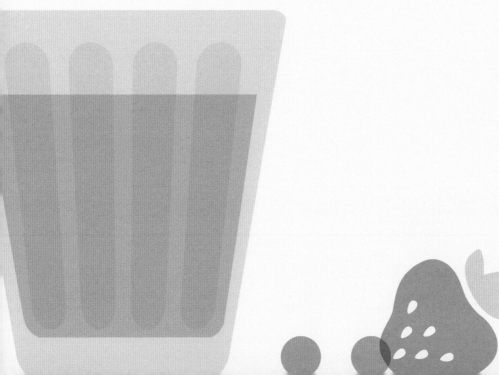

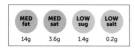

1

ENERGY 193kcals **PROTEIN** 12g | **FAT** 14g | **SATURATED FAT** 3.6g
CARBOHYDRATE 6.6g | **TOTAL SUGARS** 1.4g | **SALT** 0.2g | **SODIUM** 94mg | **FIBRE** 4.3g

Avocado & Pea Smash-up

Avocado on toast is so popular on menus everywhere that
I had to include a version of it. This avocado smash combination
can go on toast with rocket, some sliced tomato and a splash
of balsamic vinegar, plus a sprinkle of chilli flakes. Add a
handful of baby spinach leaves to boost your greens. Any
leftovers can make a dip for lunch snacking with veggies.

Serves 4

PREPARATION TIME: 15 minutes
COOKING TIME: 5 minutes

200g peas (or petits pois)
1 ripe avocado
1 tablespoon lime or lemon juice
1 small garlic clove, crushed
a small handful of mint or basil leaves
freshly ground black pepper
chilli flakes, to serve

Boil the peas for about 5 minutes, then drain well so they are fairly dry.

Spoon out the flesh of the avocado into a mini food-processor or blender and then add all the remaining ingredients, including the boiled peas. Process in pulses until you have a rough purée, scraping the sides down a couple of times. Taste and season with more lemon juice to your taste.

Cook's Tips
Try spooning some of the purée onto a plate and top with a poached or boiled egg. Asparagus would be lovely, in season.

Nutrition Tip
Avocados are a good source of soluble fibre, minerals such as iron, copper and potassium, and of vitamin E and the B vitamin, folate.

MED fat 5.7g	LOW sat 1.6g	LOW sug 2g	LOW salt 0.25g

ENERGY 101kcals **PROTEIN** 11g | **FAT** 5.7g | **SATURATED FAT** 1.6g
CARBOHYDRATE 2g | **TOTAL SUGARS** 2g | **SALT** 0.25g | **SODIUM** 107mg | **FIBRE** 0.5g

Baked Green Eggy Pots

GF

Little pots of egg for breakfast: baked to reduce the added fat in cooking and packed with protein. Try different combinations of herbs like chives or chopped peppers instead of tomatoes.

Serves 2

PREPARATION TIME: 5 minutes
COOKING TIME: 15–20 minutes

4 sprays 1-calorie sunflower oil
   cooking spray (see tip)
30g baby spinach leaves
   (or regular, roughly chopped)
2 teaspoons 0%-fat unsweetened
   Greek-style yogurt
4 cherry tomatoes (60g), halved
a few basil leaves, roughly chopped
2 eggs
freshly ground black pepper

Preheat the oven to 180°C/160°C fan/gas mark 4.

Spray two wide, ovenproof ramekin dishes with the oil and place on a baking tray. Line the ramekins with the spinach leaves. Add a blob of yogurt and then the tomatoes and basil. Crack an egg on top of each and season with pepper.

Bake in the oven for 15–20 minutes, depending on how you like your eggs.

Cook's Tip

A little spray bottle of vegetable oil is very handy, but if you don't have one, just use a few drops (⅛ teaspoon) rapeseed oil, to avoid the egg and spinach sticking to the pot.

Eating protein for breakfast is great for keeping you satisfied and making you less likely to reach for a snack before lunch.

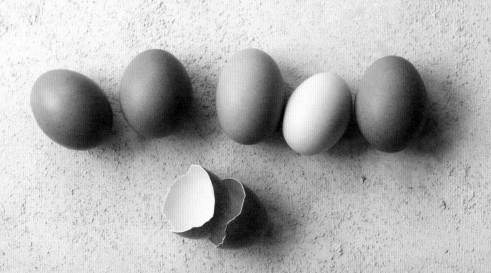

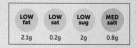

LOW fat 2.1g | LOW sat 0.2g | LOW sug 2g | MED salt 0.8g

ENERGY 134kcals **PROTEIN** 6.1g | **FAT** 2.1g | **SATURATED FAT** 0.2g
CARBOHYDRATE 23g | **TOTAL SUGARS** 2g | **SALT** 0.8g | **SODIUM** 306mg | **FIBRE** 4.5g

Creamy Mushrooms on Sourdough Toast

You can use basic button mushrooms for this or mix it up with others, such as chestnut (brown cap) mushrooms and larger, more mature portobellos. A simple recipe and full of umami flavour.

Serves 4

PREPARATION TIME: 10 minutes
COOKING TIME: 10 minutes

1 teaspoon rapeseed oil
1 small red onion (50g), finely chopped
1 garlic clove, crushed
250g mushrooms, sliced
1 teaspoon fresh lemon thyme, chopped
finely grated zest of 1 unwaxed lemon
2 tablespoons (30g) 0%-fat unsweetened Greek-style yogurt

TO SERVE
4 slices of wholemeal sourdough
a handful of fresh flat-leaf parsley, finely chopped
freshly ground black pepper

Heat the oil in a large pan and fry the onion and garlic over a medium heat for 1–2 minutes, until softened. Add the mushrooms and cook over a fairly high heat, stirring constantly, for 5–8 minutes until they brown and any liquid has evaporated.

Combine the thyme, lemon zest and yogurt in a small bowl.

Remove the mushrooms from the heat, then stir in the yogurt mixture to coat.

Toast the bread and top with the hot mushrooms, some chopped parsley and a grinding of black pepper.

Cook's Tip
Wilted baby spinach leaves would be just perfect to have with this. The mushrooms are also good as a pasta sauce, to serve two.

Nutrition Tip
Mushrooms can be a source of vitamin D, which helps the body absorb calcium.

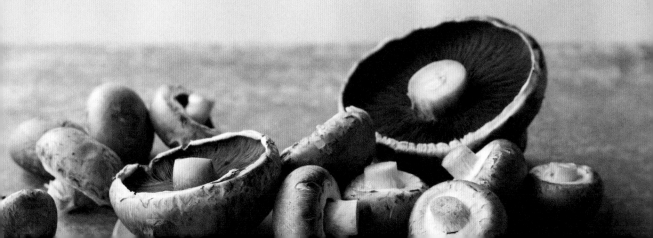

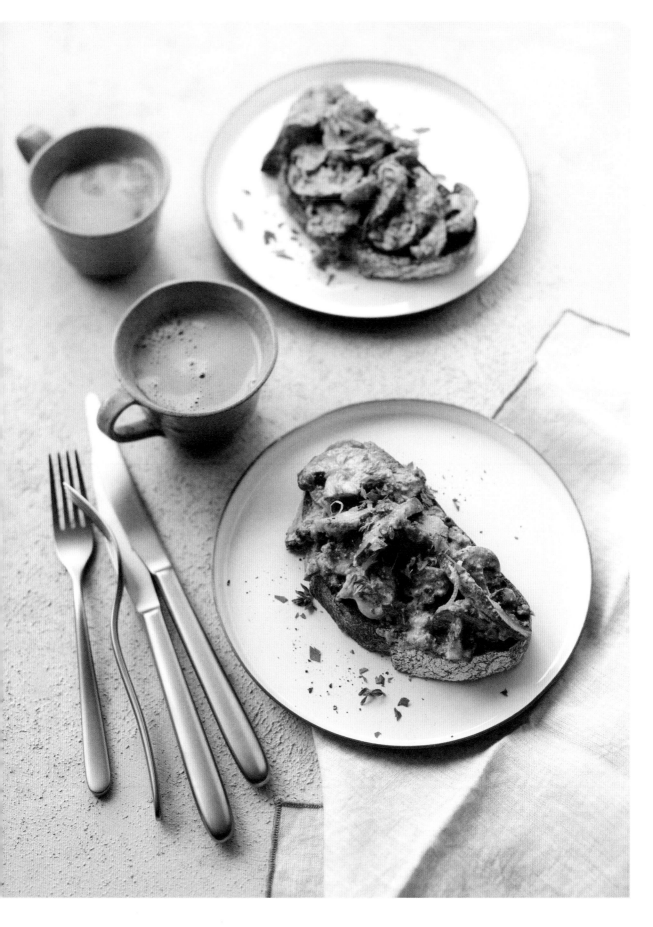

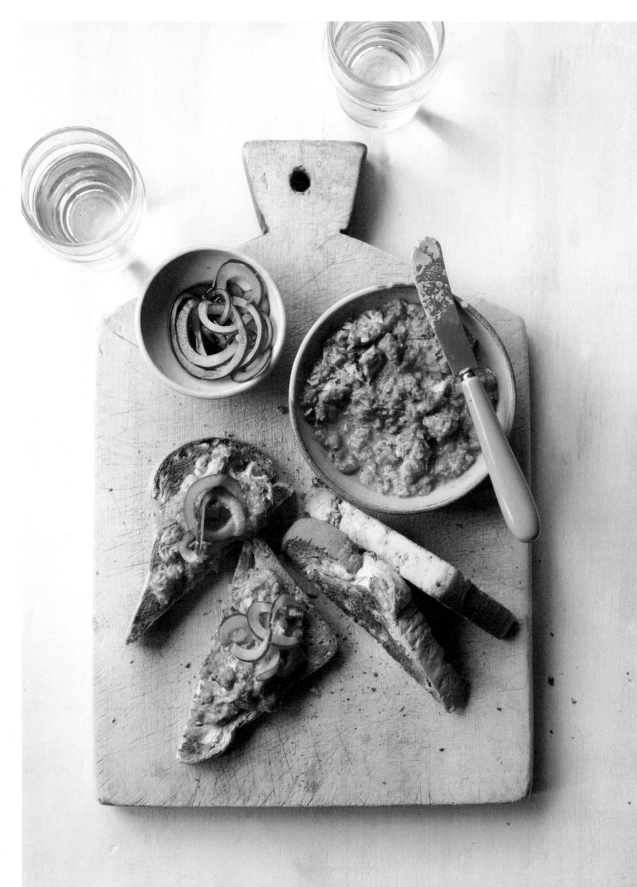

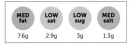

ENERGY 196kcals **PROTEIN** 10g | **FAT** 7.6g | **SATURATED FAT** 2.9g
CARBOHYDRATE 23g | **TOTAL SUGARS** 3g | **SALT** 1.3g | **SODIUM** 573mg | **FIBRE** 4.7g

Roasted Red Pepper & Sardines on Toast

This old classic of sardines on toast, in combination with sweet red peppers and seasonings, is simply delicious. You could use a jar of red peppers (in water) for ease, but it is much better to roast your own. Roasting preserves the flavour and the nutrients in the peppers as it is a dry cooking method. Keep a batch of roasted peppers in the freezer for other recipes, like this one.

Serves 4

PREPARATION TIME: 10 minutes

1 small red onion, very thinly sliced
2 teaspoons balsamic vinegar
105g can sardines in water, drained

FOR THE PEPPER PURÉE
320g roasted red peppers, roughly
    chopped
1 small garlic clove, crushed
1 tablespoon 0%-fat unsweetened
    Greek-style yogurt
¼ teaspoon sweet or smoked
    (spicy) paprika

TO SERVE
2 slices of seeded wholegrain bread
freshly ground black pepper

Place the thinly sliced red onion into a small bowl with the vinegar and set aside to pickle slightly (they taste even better if you can leave them to marinate for longer).

Remove the sardines from the can and blot any excess water on kitchen paper.

Place all of the ingredients for the pepper purée, and most of the onion slices, into a food-processor (or use a stick blender) and blend until chunky or smooth, as you prefer. Mash the sardines and stir into the pepper mixture.

To serve, toast the bread and spread with the sardine and red pepper purée. Add a few of the remaining slices of onion and a little black pepper to season.

Nutrition Tip

Canned sardines are inexpensive; they are a great source of calcium, as well as protein, and a top up for your diet of omega-3 from the oily fish.

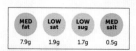

MED fat	LOW sat	LOW sug	MED salt
7.9g	1.9g	1.7g	0.5g

ENERGY 175kcals **PROTEIN** 9.4g | **FAT** 7.9g | **SATURATED FAT** 1.9g
CARBOHYDRATE 18g | **TOTAL SUGARS** 1.7g | **SALT** 0.5g | **SODIUM** 207mg | **FIBRE** 4.5g

Egg Salad on Toast

Swap the mayonnaise in a classic egg salad and use mashed avocado instead. Spread on a slice of wholemeal bread for a filling breakfast or lunch. Instead of the bread, this is also good served in a lettuce 'cup' (something like Little Gem, separated into leaves works well), which will reduce the calories, carbohydrate and fibre.

Serves 4

PREPARATION TIME: 10 minutes
COOKING TIME: 8–10 minutes

½ ripe avocado
1 teaspoon lemon juice
125g cucumber, finely chopped
a few drops chilli sauce
2 hard-boiled eggs, peeled and
   roughly chopped

TO SERVE
120g lettuce or other salad leaves
2 slices of wholemeal bread
a few chives (optional)
freshly ground black pepper

Mash the flesh from the avocado in a small bowl and add the lemon juice, chopped cucumber and chilli sauce. Mix in the hard-boiled eggs.

To serve, toast the bread and spread the avocado mixture on top, add some torn lettuce leaves, then season with pepper and snip a few chives on top, if you happen to have some.

Cook's Tip

Add more salad vegetables to the mix, chopped up small, such as red pepper or tomatoes.

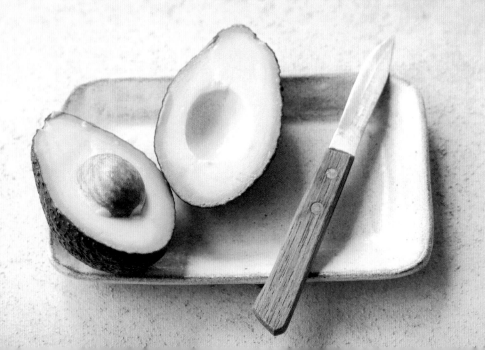

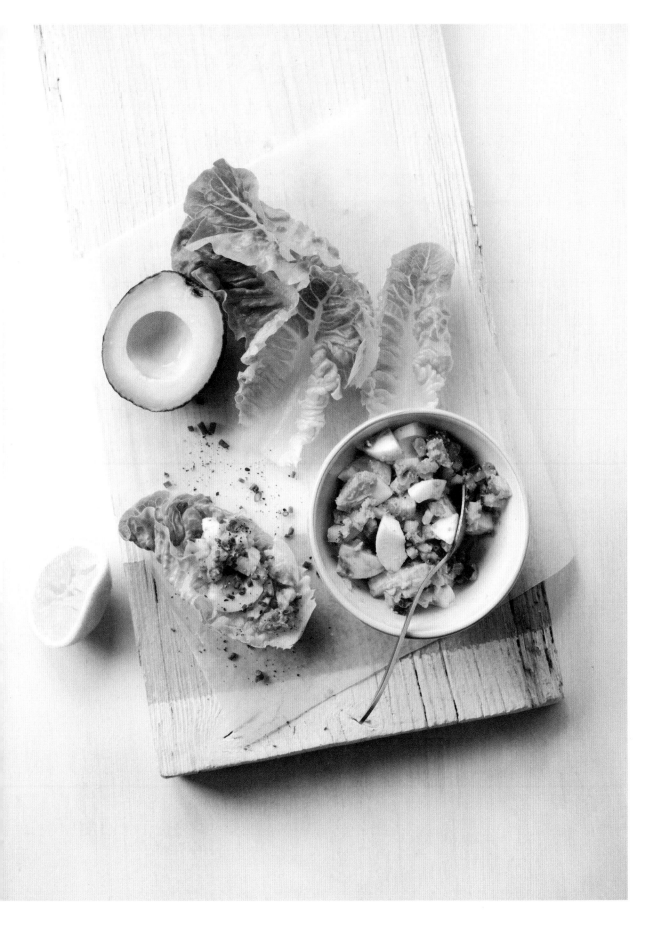

Rock & Roller Granola

Not everyone can sit down to a slow breakfast in the mornings, and you might not have much of an appetite before the commute. Here's a liquid option for those sorts of days when you're ready to rock and roll. If you like granola or muesli, why not make your own with less sugar and lots of the good stuff?

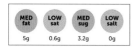

ENERGY 115kcals **PROTEIN** 3.6g | **FAT** 5g
SATURATED FAT 0.6g | **CARBOHYDRATE** 15g
TOTAL SUGARS 3.2 | **SALT** 0g | **SODIUM** 4mg | **FIBRE** 2.5g

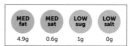

ENERGY 105kcals **PROTEIN** 3g | **FAT** 4.9g
SATURATED FAT 0.6g | **CARBOHYDRATE** 12g
TOTAL SUGARS 1g | **SALT** 0g | **SODIUM** 0mg | **FIBRE** 2.4g

---

Rock & Roller

If using
gluten-
free oats

Serves 1

PREPARATION TIME: 5 minutes

75ml cold skimmed milk
100g (1 small) banana, cut into chunks
1 tablespoon homemade granola (see right), or use shop-bought low-sugar and -salt version

Place all the ingredients into a blender and blitz until slightly smooth.

Cook's Tip
As an option, chunks of banana can be kept, wrapped, in the freezer, ready to use from frozen and put straight into the blender. Frozen fruit will chill and thicken the whole drink in an instant.

Skinny Granola

If using
gluten-
free oats

Makes 10 x 25g portions

PREPARATION TIME: 10 minutes, plus cooling
COOKING TIME: 5 minutes

175g jumbo porridge oats (or, even better, use a mixture of buckwheat flakes and oats)
15g oat bran
20g mixed seeds (such as flax, shelled hemp, pumpkin, sunflower or amaranth seeds)
3 tablespoons (30g) mixed nuts (such as walnuts, almonds and brazil nuts)
2 teaspoons runny honey (optional)
10 sprays 1-calorie sunflower oil cooking spray (optional)
pinch of ground cinnamon

Preheat the oven to 180°C/gas mark 4.

Spread out the oats, oat bran, seeds and nuts on a large, non-stick baking tray, sprinkle over the honey and oil, if using, and tumble together.

Bake for about 15 minutes, or until turning golden brown, turning the mixture every 5 minutes or so. (Don't walk too far away, as the mixture can burn easily.) Remove from the oven and leave to cool completely on the baking tray.

Stir in the cinnamon and mix together well. Store in a clean, airtight container for up to 2 months.

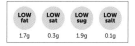
ENERGY 91kcals **PROTEIN** 4.2g | **FAT** 1.7g | **SATURATED FAT** 0.3g
CARBOHYDRATE 15g | **TOTAL SUGARS** 1.9g | **SALT** 0.1g | **SODIUM** 0mg | **FIBRE** 5.2g

Two Grain Porridge

GF
If using gluten-free oats

You could just make porridge with oats, but a great variety of other breakfast grains have become available, and it adds a healthy variation to try something new like buckwheat. You can mix it up with quinoa flakes for extra protein, too.

Use the large-flaked, whole porridge oats rather than the powdery 'instant' oat variety: The grains are less processed and slower to release energy. This power porridge helps you to feel fuller, plus the fibre found in oats, beta-glucan, is linked to lowering cholesterol.

Serves 2

PREPARATION TIME: 5 minutes
COOKING TIME: 5 minutes

20g rolled porridge oats
20g buckwheat flakes
20g oat bran
50ml skimmed milk
1 teaspoon granulated sweetener
     (optional)

Place the oats, buckwheat and oat bran into a small bowl with 400ml of water and heat in the microwave on high, for 2–3 minutes. Alternatively, on the hob, place in a small saucepan and heat to a simmer. Cook for a few minutes, adding a little more water if it thickens too much. Pour the skimmed milk over to serve and add the sweetener, if you like.

Cook's Tip

Toppings – for two servings, choose one of the following (nutrition per portion):

• 20g mixed seeds, toasted – sunflower, pumpkin or flaxseeds (57 kcals, 2.2g protein, 4.6g fat, 0.7g sat fat, 1.7g carbs, 0.2g total sugars)

• 1 tablespoon ground mixed seeds or nuts and 2 soft dates, chopped (97 kcals, 2.3g protein, 3.6g fat, 0.5g sat fat, 15g carbs, 14g total sugars)

• 20g flaked nuts – almonds, hazelnuts or mixed (46 kcals, 1.6g protein, 4.2g fat, 0.4g sat fat, 0.5g carbs, 0.3g total sugars)

• 160g frozen mixed berries, defrosted (23 kcals, 0.7g protein, 0g fat, 0g sat fat, 5g carbs, 5g total sugars)

• zest of ½ orange and segments from 1 orange (27 kcals, 0.6g protein, 0g fat, 0g sat fat, 6g carbs, 6g total sugars)

MED fat 6.8g	LOW sat 1.6g	MED sug 9.8g	LOW salt 0.1g	ENERGY 221kcals **PROTEIN** 11g | **FAT** 6.8g | **SATURATED FAT** 1.6g

ENERGY 221kcals **PROTEIN** 11g | **FAT** 6.8g | **SATURATED FAT** 1.6g
CARBOHYDRATE 28g | **TOTAL SUGARS** 9.8g | **SALT** 0.1g | **SODIUM** 47mg | **FIBRE** 7.6g

Oat & Chia Breakfast Pots

GF

If using gluten-free oats

A variation on the popular overnight oats, ready to eat in
the morning. Use the large-flaked, whole porridge oats
rather than the powdery 'instant' oat variety: they are less
processed and slower to release energy. The jumbo oats will
also keep their texture well overnight, so the result is less
gluey than instant porridge.

Serves 1

PREPARATION TIME: 5 minutes, plus
refrigeration overnight

30g rolled porridge oats
2 teaspoons chia seeds
100ml skimmed milk or
    almond milk
1 teaspoon unsweetened
    cocoa powder
granulated sweetener (optional)
50g blueberries or blackberries,
    to serve

Mix all the ingredients together in a clean jar or bowl, cover and leave
in the fridge overnight.

Serve with some blueberries or blackberries.

Nutrition Tip
Chia seeds are an excellent source of plant proteins and fibre; the
soluble type of fibre found in oats (beta-glucan) can help to lower
cholesterol and is associated with a reduced risk of heart disease.

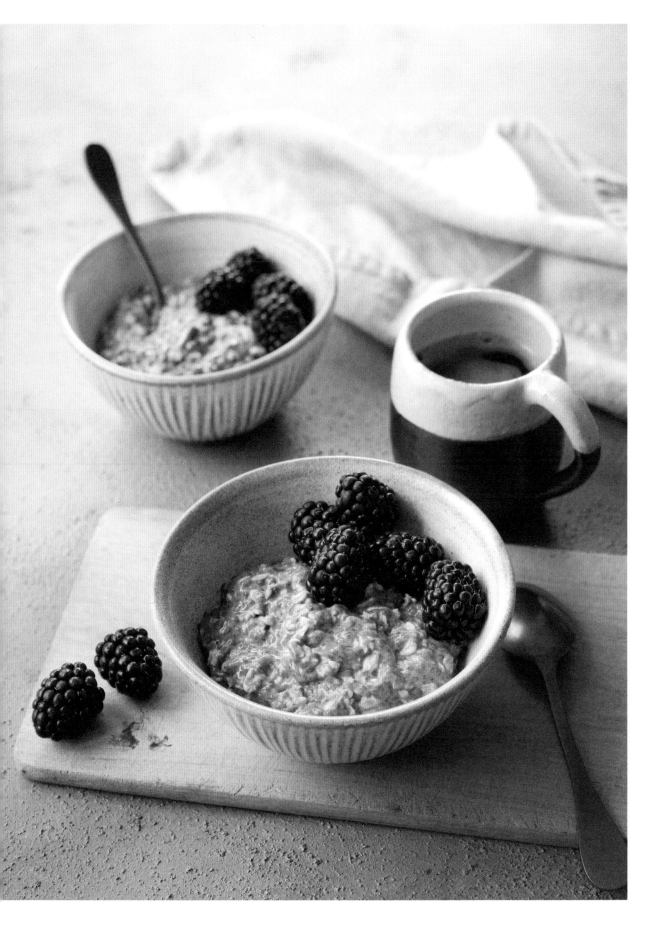

Power Smoothies

Straight juicing is a fast option but can take most of the fibre goodness out of the fruit and vegetables, leaving just a sugary drink; so, proceed with caution and limit the total amount of fruit juice or smoothie you have to just one small glass, 150ml, a day. If you do opt for a smoothie, add some fibre and a boost of nutrients in the ingredients you choose, to contribute to your daily dose of greens.

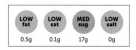

LOW fat	LOW sat	MED sug	LOW salt
0.5g	0.1g	17g	0g

ENERGY 80kcals **PROTEIN** 1.7g | **FAT** 0.5g
SATURATED FAT 0.1g | **CARBOHYDRATE** 18g
TOTAL SUGARS 17g | **SALT** 0g | **SODIUM** 13mg | **FIBRE** 3.5g

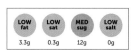

LOW fat	LOW sat	MED sug	LOW salt
3.3g	0.3g	12g	0g

ENERGY 116kcals **PROTEIN** 3.7g | **FAT** 3.3g
SATURATED FAT 0.3g | **CARBOHYDRATE** 18g
TOTAL SUGARS 12g | **SALT** 0g | **SODIUM** 13mg | **FIBRE** 3.3g

The Green One

Serves 1

PREPARATION TIME: 5 minutes

½ small banana, peeled and cut into chunks
80g (1 small) pear, chopped (skin on)
20g kale leaves, chopped and tough stems removed
75ml water
1 tablespoon lemon juice
1 heaped teaspoon peeled and grated fresh ginger (optional)
ice cubes, to serve (optional)

Place all the ingredients in a food-processor or blender. Pulse a few times and then purée until almost smooth, scraping down the sides as necessary. It will be nice and thick but, of course, add more water until it is the right consistency for you.

Cook's Tip
I'm singing the praises of the freezer here, to keep some washed and chopped kale, frozen and ready to use.

The Super Green & Wholesome One

Serves 1

PREPARATION TIME: 5 minutes

½ small banana, cut into chunks
juice of 1 lime
20g spinach leaves, chopped and tough stems removed
20g broccoli florets, stems removed
35ml pressed cloudy apple juice
1 teaspoon milled flaxseeds (optional)
ice cubes, to serve (optional)

Try this: it tastes surprisingly good! Place all the ingredients in a food-processor or blender with 40ml water. Pulse a few times and then purée until almost smooth, scraping down the sides as necessary. Adding ground flaxseeds will make it thicker, so add a little water until it is the right consistency for you.

Cook's Tip
Purple sprouting broccoli tops would be great in here, if you happen to have some.

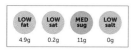

ENERGY 132kcals **PROTEIN** 6.5g | **FAT** 4.9g
SATURATED FAT 0.2g | **CARBOHYDRATE** 12g
TOTAL SUGARS 11g | **SALT** 0g | **SODIUM** 0mg | **FIBRE** 3.2g

The Dairy Berry One

Serves 1

PREPARATION TIME: 5 minutes

100g low-fat, unsweetened live yogurt or kefir
80g frozen mixed berries and currants (i.e. summer
    fruits, forest fruits)
1 teaspoon milled flaxseeds
granulated sweetener, to taste (optional)

Blend the yogurt, berries and flaxseeds in a blender
until smooth. A stick bender in a tall jug is easiest
for making single smoothies. Add sweetener to
taste, if using, and serve.

Cook's Tip

If you use frozen fruit then the result will be thick
and refreshingly ice cold, and you'll probably need
to eat it with a spoon. If you want more of a drink,
defrost the fruit first, or you can make it with fresh
fruit, of course. Blackcurrants and red currants can
be a little tart: add a touch of sweetener if it's too
sharp for you.

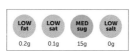

ENERGY 68kcals **PROTEIN** 1.8g | **FAT** 0.2g
SATURATED FAT 0.1g | **CARBOHYDRATE** 16g
TOTAL SUGARS 15g | **SALT** 0g | **SODIUM** 11mg | **FIBRE** 1.2g

The Fruity Ice Cream One

Okay, this is not a smoothie at all: it's a cheat's
ice cream and I would have it for pudding.
Delicious made with any frozen mixed fruit
and healthier than ice cream anyway.

Makes 200g or 4 small scoops (serves 2)

PREPARATION TIME: 5 minutes

80g frozen dark cherries
1 small banana (100g), cut into chunks and frozen
50ml skimmed milk

Place all the ingredients into a blender and blitz
until smooth but still with some chunks of fruit.

Cook's Tip
Banana is a magic ingredient for sweetening and
thickening that can be conveniently kept in the
freezer ready to use from frozen. Buy small ones,
not too ripe.

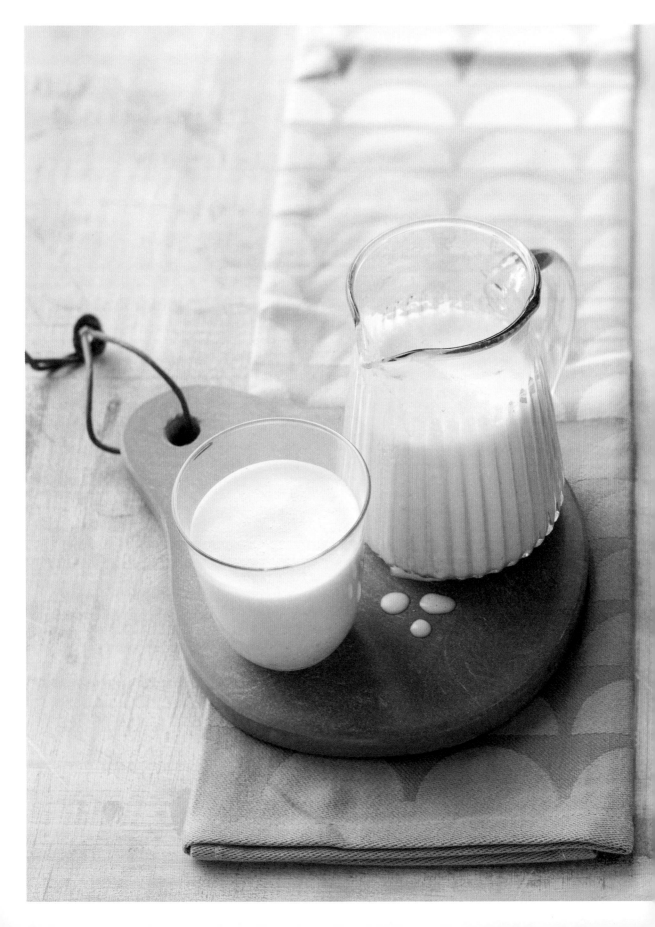

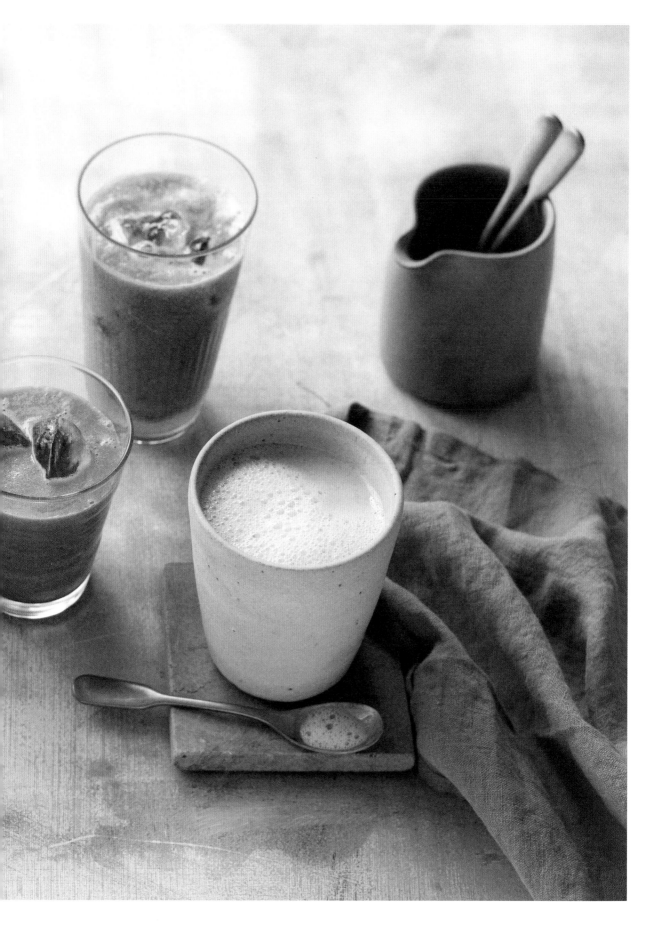

Fresh Almond Milk Drinks

Making your own nut milk is simple and you can keep it in a container in the fridge for a few days, to enjoy warmed or cold. It contains nothing more than fresh almonds and filtered water. No additives needed. The characteristics of almond milk complement coffee well.

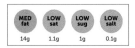

ENERGY 153kcals **PROTEIN** 0.5g | **FAT** 14g
SATURATED FAT 1.1g | **CARBOHYDRATE** 1.7g
TOTAL SUGARS 1g | **SALT** 0.1g | **SODIUM** 8.5mg | **FIBRE** 2.5g

---

Almond Milk

Ve GF

Serves 4 (makes approx. 500ml)

PREPARATION TIME: 10 minutes, plus soaking overnight

100g almonds (skin on), soaked overnight in water
500ml filtered or mineral water, plus extra for
   soaking overnight

Drain the soaked nuts, then place in a blender with 200ml of the filtered or mineral water. Blend until almost smooth. Add the remaining 300ml of water and blend again to mix. Strain through a fine mesh sieve into a jug and discard the solid grainy bits.

Store the liquid in a sterilised, airtight jar or sealed container in the fridge. Use within 5 days. The liquid will separate in the fridge, so stir before using.

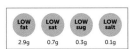

ENERGY 127kcals **PROTEIN** 2.7g | **FAT** 2.9g
SATURATED FAT 0.7g | **CARBOHYDRATE** 0.2g
TOTAL SUGARS 0.3g | **SALT** 0.1g | **SODIUM** 53mg | **FIBRE** 1g

---

Almond Milk Latte

Ve GF

Great for a morning coffee break, or chill it down for an iced summer drink.

Serves 1

PREPARATION TIME: 5 minutes

125ml almond milk (see left)
1 shot freshly brewed espresso

Heat a small cupful of almond milk. Froth it up and add the shot of espresso.

Nutrition Tip

Dairy products contain essential nutrients that nut milks do not, such as calcium, protein, vitamin B12 and iodine. If you are switching from cow's milk, ensure you include plenty of alternative sources like bony fish (tinned salmon, sardines, whitebait), calcium-enriched tofu, green leafy vegetables like broccoli and cabbage (not spinach), beans and sesame seeds.

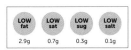

2.9g 0.7g 0.3g 0.1g

ENERGY 127kcals **PROTEIN** 2.7g | **FAT** 2.9g
SATURATED FAT 0.7g | **CARBOHYDRATE** 0.2g
TOTAL SUGARS 0.3g | **SALT** 0.1g | **SODIUM** 53mg | **FIBRE** 1g

Turmeric Latte

If you have a sense of food adventure and a willingness to try something new, add some warming spices.

Serves 1

PREPARATION TIME: 5 minutes

125ml almond milk
pinch of ground turmeric
pinch of ground cinnamon
½ teaspoon vanilla extract or sprinkle of sweetener
   (optional)

Warm all the ingredients together and pour into a cup to serve. If you like to sweeten your milk, then add the vanilla extract or a sprinkle of sweetener granules.

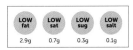

2.9g 0.7g 0.3g 0.1g

ENERGY 127kcals **PROTEIN** 2.7g | **FAT** 2.9g
SATURATED FAT 0.7g | **CARBOHYDRATE** 0.2g
TOTAL SUGARS 0.3g | **SALT** 0.1g | **SODIUM** 53mg | **FIBRE** 1g

Chai-style Latte

Not just for tea – chai flavour compliments almond milk well.

Serves 1

PREPARATION TIME: 5 minutes

125ml almond milk
chai-flavour tea bag

Warm the almond milk and pour into a cup. Place a chai-flavour tea bag in the warm milk for a chai-style flavour.

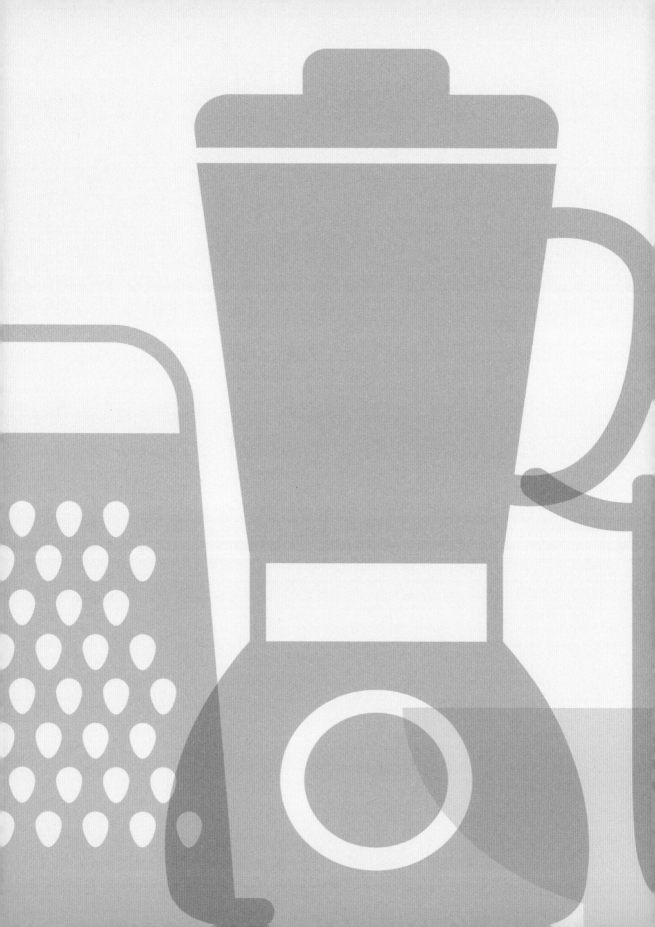

Satisfying Soups

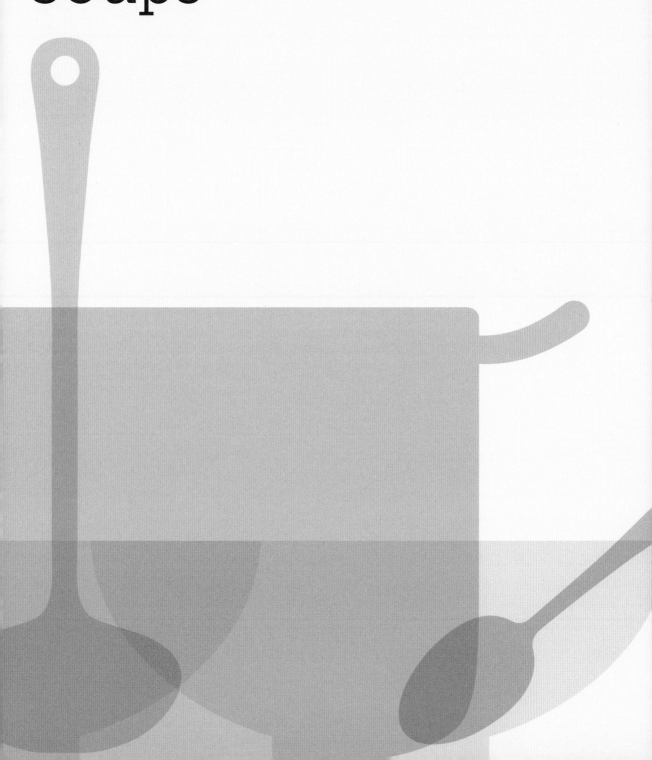

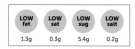

2

ENERGY 67kcals **PROTEIN** 4.7g | **FAT** 1.3g | **SATURATED FAT** 0.3g
CARBOHYDRATE 9.6g | **TOTAL SUGARS** 5.4g | **SALT** 0.2g | **SODIUM** 141mg | **FIBRE** 5.1g·

Herb Broth with Spring Onions & Ginger

If using gluten-free stock cube

A cleansing, tasty, simple soup that you can make and leave in the fridge until needed. I sometimes even eat it cold. The flavour here is from the herbs and ginger.

Serves 4

PREPARATION TIME: 10 minutes
COOKING TIME: 10–15 minutes

10g reduced-salt vegetable stock cube
8 spring onions, thinly sliced on an angle
2 tablespoons chopped fresh ginger
2 medium carrots, peeled and cut into small cubes
2 courgettes, chopped into small cubes
150g frozen peas
4 heaped tablespoons each freshly chopped parsley, tarragon, basil and coriander
freshly ground black pepper

Place 1 litre of water into a small saucepan with the stock cube, spring onions, ginger and carrots and bring to the boil. Turn down the heat and simmer gently for 15 minutes.

Next add the courgettes and peas and bring back to just a simmer. Remove from the heat and add the herbs and pepper. Serve piping hot straight away or allow to cool and store in the fridge for 3–4 days or in the freezer for 1 month.

Nutrition Tip

This recipe is packed with nutritious vegetables. Carrots are packed with beta-carotene, which converts into vitamin A when eaten. Both peas and ginger can have anti-inflammatory properties, and ginger can promote good gastro-intestinal health.

LOW fat	LOW sat	LOW sug	MED salt
2g	0.4g	2.4g	0.3g

ENERGY 194kcals **PROTEIN** 21g | **FAT** 2g | **SATURATED FAT** 0.4g
CARBOHYDRATE 23g | **TOTAL SUGARS** 2.4g | **SALT** 0.3g | **SODIUM** 126mg | **FIBRE** 4.5g

Simple Turkey & Mushroom Broth

GF
If using gluten-free miso paste

I love this dish: so simple but really tasty. The only oil I use is a little sesame oil to flavour the end dish. I do not add salt and rely on fish sauce and the miso sachet to give the needed background flavour.

Serves 4

PREPARATION TIME: 20 minutes
COOKING TIME: 15 minutes

250g turkey breast mince (skinless)
15g sachet miso soup paste
8 spring onions, very finely sliced, plus extra to serve
250g chestnut or open cap mushrooms, finely sliced
250g green beans, chopped into 1cm pieces
½ teaspoon sesame oil
½ teaspoon fish sauce
150g fresh baby spinach leaves
100g cooked wholegrain rice vermicelli
fresh red chilli, sliced
freshly ground black pepper

Place roughly 800ml of cold water into a pan with the turkey mince and break up with a wooden spoon. Squeeze the miso paste into the pan and mix well, then add the spring onions and mushrooms and mix well again. Place over a medium heat until simmering, then cook for 10 minutes.

Add the beans and cook for 5 minutes, then add the oil, fish sauce and pepper to taste.

To serve, place the spinach and cooked rice vermicelli into four bowls, then ladle the broth over equally. Serve with a little extra sliced spring onion and some sliced red chilli.

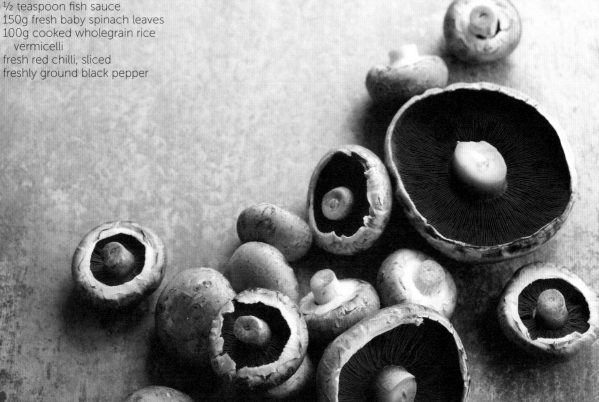

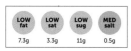

ENERGY 215kcals PROTEIN 16g | FAT 7.3g | SATURATED FAT 3.3g
CARBOHYDRATE 22g | TOTAL SUGARS 11g | SALT 0.5g | SODIUM 215mg | FIBRE 10g

Minestrone Greens & Beans

Ve
If omitting
parmesan

GF
If using
gluten-
free stock
cubes and
miso paste

This is a hearty mixed vegetable soup that will satisfy and it's
easily adaptable to use 'what's-in-the-fridge' vegetables. I'm
using beans instead of potatoes and you can switch in any mix
of beans. I've tweaked in a tiny bit of miso paste to make the
flavour sing; feel free to play around with herbs and spices, too.
If you have time to simmer this pot for longer than 30 minutes,
the vegetables will be softer and taste even better.

Serves 4

PREPARATION TIME: 15 minutes
COOKING TIME: 40 minutes

1 teaspoon rapeseed oil
1 large red onion, finely chopped
2 garlic cloves, chopped
1 medium carrot, peeled and cut
　into small dice
1 celery stick, trimmed and thinly
　sliced
1 courgette, cut into small dice
200g mushrooms
400g can chopped tomatoes
500ml reduced-salt vegetable or
　chicken stock
1 teaspoon dried Italian mixed
　herbs or oregano
1 teaspoon miso paste (optional)
400g can cannellini beans, drained
　and rinsed
200g spinach, washed, chopped
　and tough stalks removed
a handful of fresh basil leaves
a handful of flat-leaf parsley, finely
　chopped

TO SERVE (OPTIONAL)
4 teaspoons grated Parmesan
freshly ground black pepper

Heat the oil in a large saucepan over a fairly high heat and fry the
onion, garlic, carrot, celery, courgette and mushrooms for about
10 minutes until the vegetables are soft and fragrant.

Add the tomatoes, stock, dried herbs and miso, if using, and bring to
a boil. Next add the beans, then cover and simmer for 30 minutes:
the vegetables will still have some bite and texture after this time.

Remove from the heat, stir through the spinach, basil and parsley and
allow to stand for 5 minutes. Taste and season with black pepper and
a teaspoon of cheese for each bowl, if using.

Nutrition Tip
Like all beans, cannellini contain fairly high amounts of carbohydrate,
but a significant proportion is pure fibre and they will help keep you
full for longer. They have a lower GI than potatoes and are also low in
fat and full of protein.

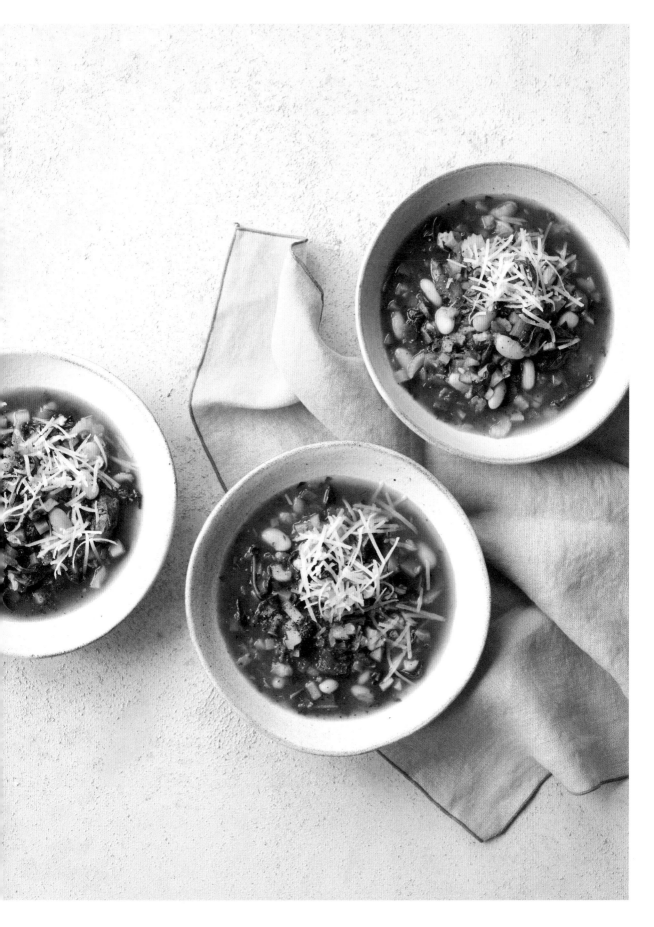

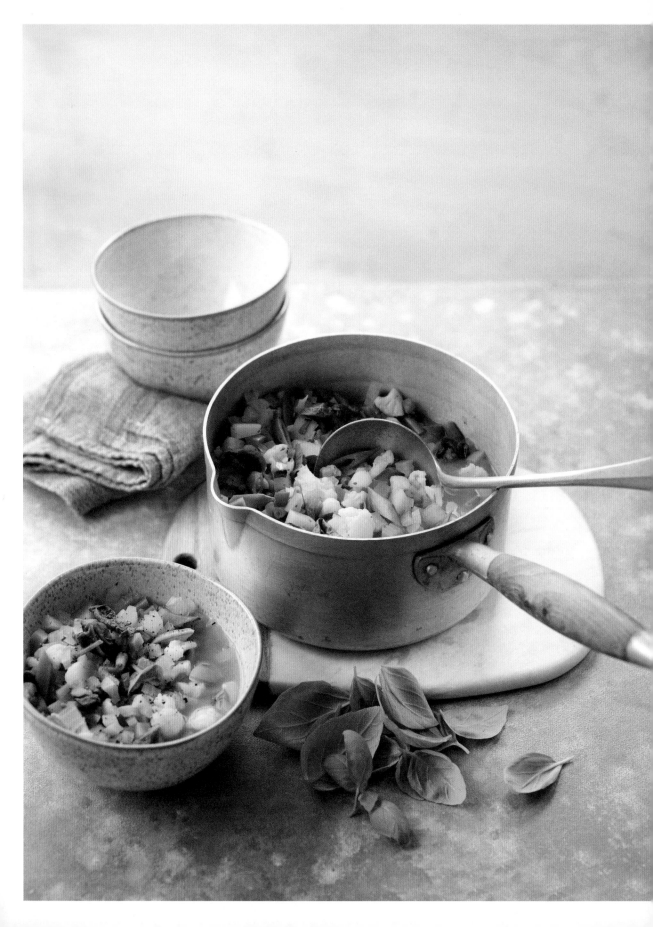

LOW fat	LOW sat	LOW sug	LOW salt
1.4g	0.2g	18g	0.2g

ENERGY 155kcals **PROTEIN** 7.7g | **FAT** 1.4g | **SATURATED FAT** 0.2g
CARBOHYDRATE 30g | **TOTAL SUGARS** 18g | **SALT** 0.2g | **SODIUM** 74mg | **FIBRE** 12g

Summer Vegetable Soup

Ve

GF

If using gluten-free stock cube

When I was training to be a chef we used to make minestrone: the golden rule, the head chef told me, was that there should be so much veg once cooked that the wooden spoon should stand up in the centre of the pot. With that in mind, try this summer soup, packed with lots of veg, plus aromatics such as ginger, lemongrass and oregano. You can add a little dried spaghetti, or even rice, to make another variation, if you really want.

Serves 4

PREPARATION TIME: 30 minutes
COOKING TIME: 25–30 minutes

2 onions, peeled and chopped
4 celery sticks, chopped
2 medium carrots, peeled and chopped
1 yellow pepper, deseeded and chopped
1 red pepper, deseeded and chopped
1 orange pepper, deseeded and chopped
2 small potatoes, peeled and chopped
10g reduced-salt vegetable stock cube
1 tablespoon lemongrass purée
1 tablespoon ginger purée
1 tablespoon dried oregano
1 small cauliflower, cut into small florets
200g green beans, chopped into 1cm pieces
200g mangetout
100g baby spinach leaves

TO SERVE
2 small bunches of fresh basil
freshly ground black pepper

Place all the vegetables up to the potato into a large saucepan along with the stock cube, lemongrass and ginger purées and oregano. Cover with approximately 1 litre of water. Bring to the boil, and then simmer for 15–20 minutes until the vegetables are just cooked.

Add the cauliflower, green beans, mangetout and baby spinach leaves and cook for a further 5 minutes.

Remove from the heat, check the seasoning and add the basil just before serving.

Nutrition Tip
Cauliflower is very low in calories and contains lots of essential vitamins and minerals.

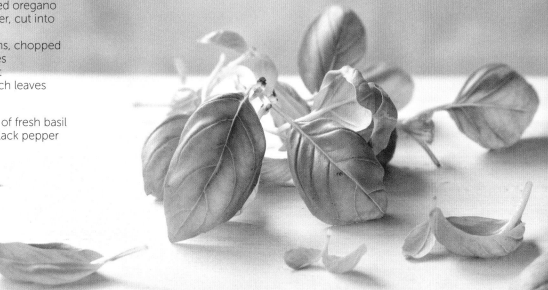

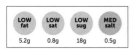

ENERGY 183kcals **PROTEIN** 6g | **FAT** 5.2g | **SATURATED FAT** 0.8g
CARBOHYDRATE 31g | **TOTAL SUGARS** 18g | **SALT** 0.5g | **SODIUM** 209mg | **FIBRE** 8g

LOW fat 5.2g | LOW sat 0.8g | LOW sug 18g | MED salt 0.5g

My Gazpacho

I know this is not a true gazpacho in its purest form, although there are many regional variations. I use canned tomatoes for ease and pack in as much veg as possible. But, it's so simple to make and it's my wife's favourite chilled soup.

Serves 4

PREPARATION TIME: 15 minutes

2 red peppers, deseeded
2 yellow peppers, deseeded
½ cucumber, peeled
400g can chopped tomatoes
  in juice
4 large tomatoes
1 onion, roughly chopped
4 garlic cloves, roughly chopped
100g (2 slices) wholemeal bread,
  roughly broken up
10g reduced-salt vegetable
  stock cube
1 tablespoon Worcester sauce
2 teaspoons Tabasco
2 tablespoons vinegar (any will
  do but I use sherry)
½ teaspoon granulated sweetener
1 tablespoon extra virgin olive oil
freshly ground black pepper

Liquidise all the vegetables, aromatics, bread and stock cube together. Add the Worcester sauce, Tabasco, vinegar and sugar, and mix well.

Finally add the olive oil and pepper in small quantities until you have the desired taste. To finish, chill well and serve in mugs, cups or glasses.

Nutrition Tip

As antioxidant-boosting veg go, peppers are pretty high on the scale. They are also great sources of fibre and vitamin C, and provide a good amount of vitamin A.

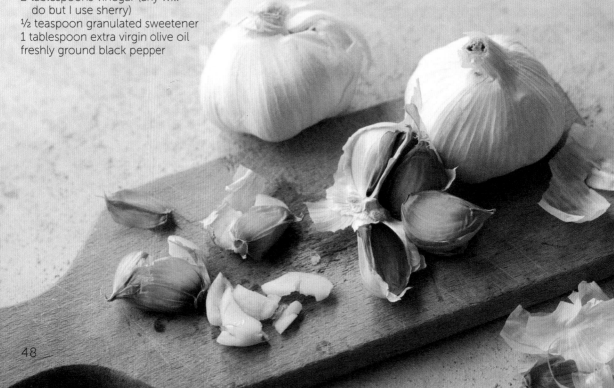

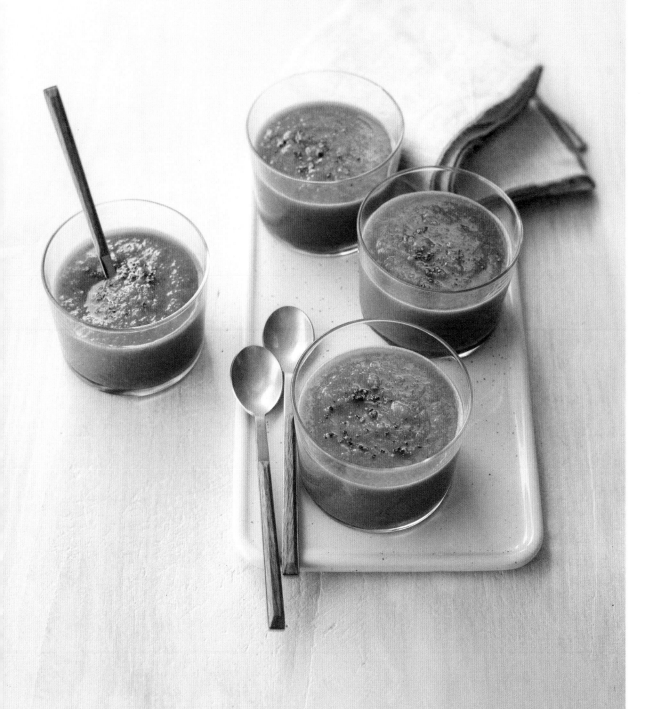

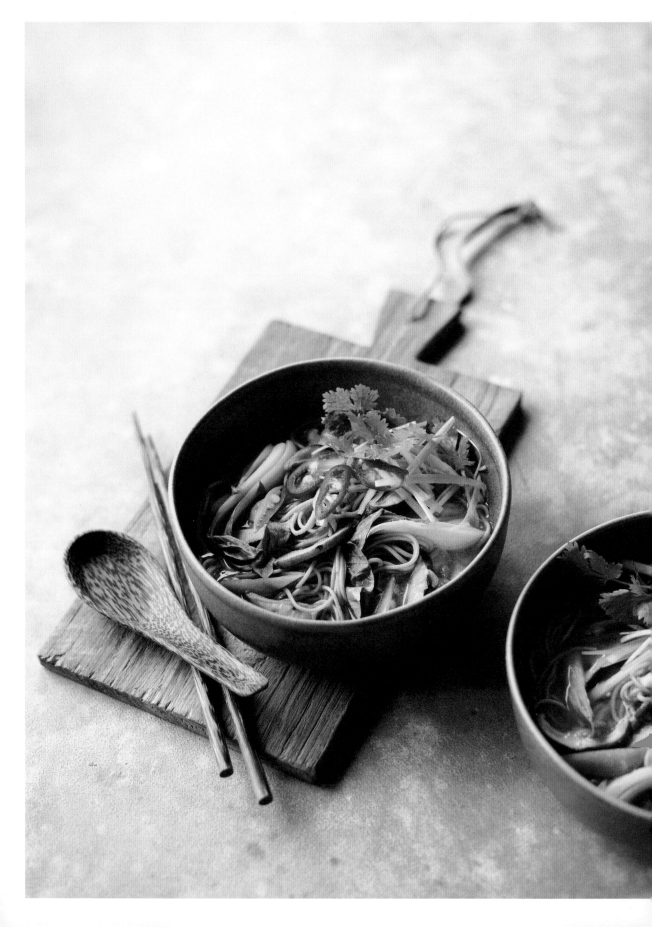

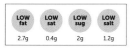

LOW fat	LOW sat	LOW sug	LOW salt
2.7g	0.4g	2g	1.2g

ENERGY 213kcals **PROTEIN** 10g | **FAT** 2.7g | **SATURATED FAT** 0.4g
CARBOHYDRATE 41g | **TOTAL SUGARS** 2g | **SALT** 1.2g | **SODIUM** 76mg | **FIBRE** 2.7g

Mixed Mushroom & Chinese Noodle Soup

Brown cap, white button, shiitake or mixed wild mushrooms: even dried mushrooms are good to use in this dish. I have also cooked this with a pack of frozen mixed wild mushrooms, because, I was surprised to find, they were cheaper. I like to keep the noodles separate from the soup as they tend to thicken it.

Serves 4

PREPARATION TIME: 15 minutes
COOKING TIME: 15 minutes

200g dried soba noodles (buckwheat)
450g mixed mushrooms
180g pak choi
10g reduced-salt vegetable stock cube dissolved in 600ml boiling water
1–2 teaspoons finely chopped or grated fresh ginger
1 teaspoon light soy sauce or 1 teaspoon miso paste
¼ teaspoon Chinese 5 spice powder
2 star anise (optional)
1 teaspoon rapeseed oil
1 onion, finely chopped
80g sugar snap peas

TO SERVE (OPTIONAL)
½ teaspoon sesame oil
2 spring onions, cut into matchsticks
a handful of fresh herbs (coriander leaves or Thai basil and mint leaves)
1 large, mild red chilli, finely sliced on the diagonal

Bring a large pot of water to the boil and cook the noodles according to the packet instructions. Keep an eye out as they like to foam up and boil over. Refresh under cold water, drain and set aside.

Wipe the mushrooms and slice thinly if using fresh ones, or rehydrate dried ones in a little boiling water, to cover (you can add this liquid into the stock for extra flavour later). Remove the core from the pak choi, cut the leaves crossways into four, then wash thoroughly and drain.

Bring the stock to the boil in a large pan. Add the ginger, soy sauce or miso, 5 spice and the star anise, if using. Reduce the heat to low and infuse while you cook the onions and mushrooms in a separate pan.

Add the oil to a large, non-stick sauté pan, then add the onion and the mushrooms and cook over a fairly high heat for 10 minutes, stirring regularly until they begin to colour. Add the hot stock to the pan with the mushrooms and bring back to a simmer. Remove the star anise, if using. Stir in the pak choi and sugar snap peas and simmer for a further 3 minutes or until the vegetables are just tender.

Remove the pan from the heat. Reheat the noodles briefly and coat in 1 teaspoon of sesame oil, if using. To serve, place a portion of noodles in a deep bowl and ladle the mushroom soup over. Put the spring onion, herbs and chilli in a separate bowl, if using and serve alongside the soup.

ENERGY 140kcals | **PROTEIN** 4.2g | **FAT** 1.2g | **SATURATED FAT** 0.3g
CARBOHYDRATE 30g | **TOTAL SUGARS** 9.5g | **SALT** 0.15g | **SODIUM** 77mg | **FIBRE** 6g

Sweet Potato & Watercress Vichyssoise

If using gluten-free stock cube

It's not everybody's cup of tea, a chilled soup, but sometimes, on a hot day, it's rather nice. Of course, you can eat this soup hot, but if you do, add the watercress at the last second to keep it fresh and crisp. The one potato helps give the finished soup and nice texture, but you can remove if you so desire. No need to sauté anything here; this also negates the use of any oil or butter, keeping the calories down.

Serves 4

PREPARATION TIME: 20 minutes
COOKING TIME: 15–20 minutes

2 onions, chopped
2 garlic cloves, crushed
3 large sweet potatoes, peeled and roughly chopped
1 large potato, peeled and roughly chopped
2 teaspoons cumin seeds
1 litre boiling water
10g reduced-salt vegetable stock cube
2 large bunches of watercress (approx. 200g)
freshly ground black pepper

Place the onions, garlic, both types of potato, cumin seeds, water and stock cube into a large saucepan and bring to the boil. Reduce to a simmer and cook for 12–15 minutes until all the potatoes are cooked.

Once the potatoes are cooked, season with a little pepper, then carefully liquidise in a blender or purée using a stick blender until you have a nice fine purée. Cool and chill well in the fridge until needed.

When ready to serve, remove the chilled soup from the fridge, check the seasoning and stir through the watercress. Serve in deep bowls.

Nutrition Tip
Watercress is low in sodium and rich in vitamins A and C, as well as being a good source of folate, calcium, iron and vitamin E.

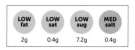

ENERGY 181kcals **PROTEIN** 22g | **FAT** 2g | **SATURATED FAT** 0.4g

CARBOHYDRATE 19g | **TOTAL SUGARS** 7.2g | **SALT** 0.4g | **SODIUM** 176mg | **FIBRE** 8.2g

Tuna Cauliflower Bean Broth

GF

If using gluten-free stock cube

Not an ingredient you would normally associate with a soup, but tuna works really well: I once had a tuna soup in Spain. Canned tuna has quite a pronounced flavour, so a little does go a long way. Just ensure you add it at the very last minute to just warm through. If using fresh tuna, place into hot bowls and pour the boiling broth over; there will be plenty of heat to just warm the tuna without overcooking it.

Serves 4

PREPARATION TIME: 10 minutes
COOKING TIME: 15 minutes

½ × 10g reduced-salt fish stock cube
1 teaspoon chopped fresh red chilli
2 onions, finely chopped
4 garlic cloves, crushed
1 medium cauliflower, broken
    into small florets, stalk cut into
    5mm cubes
420g can cannellini beans, drained
100g baby spinach leaves
juice of 2 limes
4 tablespoons fresh coriander,
    chopped
½ teaspoon toasted sesame oil
250g can tuna in water, well
    drained and flaked

Place 750ml of water with the stock cube, chilli, onions and garlic into a large pan and bring to the boil. Simmer for 10 minutes.

Next add the cauliflower and beans and cook until the cauliflower is just cooked, about 3–4 minutes.

Finally, add the spinach and wilt, then add the lime juice, coriander, sesame oil and finally the flaked tuna. Serve.

Nutrition Tip
Cauliflower is surprisingly high in vitamin C and folic acid. To reduce the amount of salt in this recipe, you can omit the stock cube.

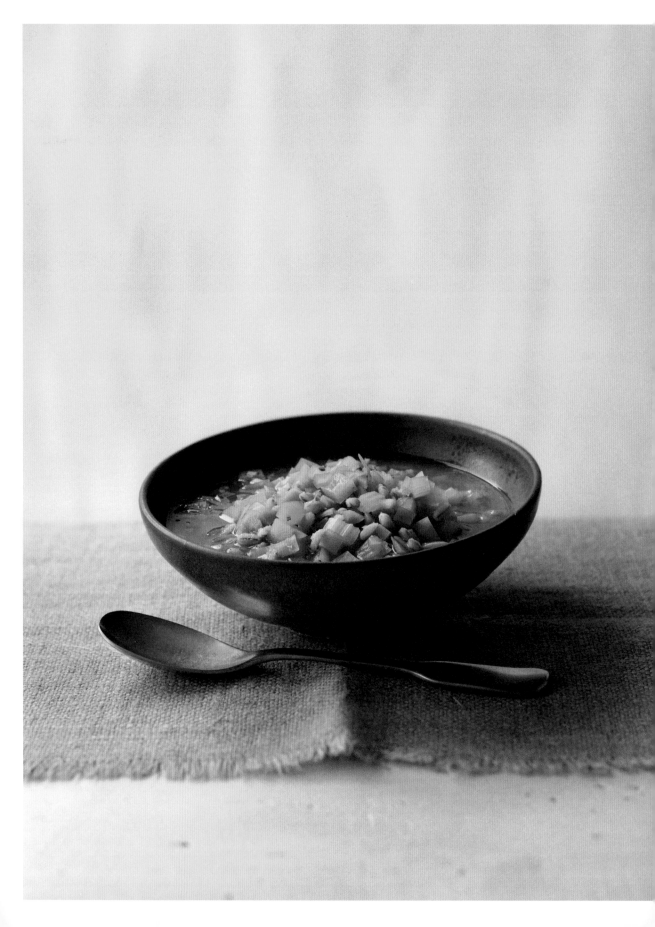

ENERGY 191kcals **PROTEIN** 48g | **FAT** 1.2g | **SATURATED FAT** 0.3g
CARBOHYDRATE 43g | **TOTAL SUGARS** 7.3g | **SALT** 0.1g | **SODIUM** 40mg | **FIBRE** 8.8g

Barley Soup with Allspice, Sage & Onion

Although this looks really simple, the end result is a warming, hearty meal. The main thing to remember is to soak the barley overnight, as it cuts down the cooking time by a huge amount. Other grains work really well such as kamut, spelt, freekeh and faro, which I soak overnight, too.

Serves 4

PREPARATION TIME: 20 minutes
COOKING TIME: 1 hour

100g pearl barley (soaked overnight)
3 small onions, finely chopped
1 small swede, peeled and finely chopped
250g waxy potatoes, finely chopped
1 medium carrot, peeled and finely chopped
1 small leek, washed well and finely chopped
2 small celery sticks, finely chopped
1 teaspoon ground allspice
2 teaspoons dried sage
10g reduced-salt vegetable stock cube
freshly ground black pepper

Place everything, yes, everything, into a saucepan with roughly 750ml of water and bring to the boil. Turn down the heat and gently simmer for 35–45 minutes, until the barley is cooked through; then everything else will also be cooked. That's it!

Nutrition Tips

One-pot cooking retains water-soluble nutrients such as B vitamins.

All types of onion can benefit digestive health as they contain inulin, which feeds the good bacteria in the gut.

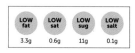

ENERGY 164kcals **PROTEIN** 6.5g | **FAT** 3.3g | **SATURATED FAT** 0.6g

CARBOHYDRATE 27g | **TOTAL SUGARS** 11g | **SALT** 0.1g | **SODIUM** 36mg | **FIBRE** 8.3g

Thick Bean and Dark Cabbage Stew

If using
gluten-
free stock
cube

This is more like a nourishing vegetable and bean stew than a soup, adapted from a traditional Tuscan style ribollita. Cavolo nero is a dark green cabbage, typical of Tuscany, but you can use kale or Savoy cabbage instead. Unlike spinach, cavolo nero needs a bit longer to cook; it is particularly good to partner with beans or lentils. The flavour seems to be better after a day or so: true to the meaning of ribollita or 're-boiled', so you can prepare it ahead and reheat it.

Serves 6

PREPARATION TIME: 15 minutes
COOKING TIME: 45 minutes

1 tablespoon olive oil
1 medium carrot, peeled and finely chopped
1 large onion (230g), finely chopped
1 celery stick, trimmed and finely chopped
1 garlic clove, crushed
350g cavolo nero, washed, trimmed and finely sliced
250g sweet potatoes, peeled and cut into small chunks
400g can borlotti beans
400g can chopped tomatoes
4–5 sprigs of fresh thyme, leaves picked, or small pinch of dried
few sprigs of rosemary
400ml reduced-salt vegetable stock
freshly ground black pepper

In a large, wide pan, heat the oil over a fairly high heat and fry the carrot, onion and celery for about 5 minutes. Add the garlic.

Remove any tough stalks from the cavolo nero and add the leaves to the vegetables in the pan along with the sweet potatoes. Sauté for a further 10 minutes, stirring.

If using canned beans, drain and rinse them well, then mash or blend half of them with a little cold water. Stir the borlotti beans (mashed and whole), into the pan and add the chopped tomatoes, fresh thyme and rosemary, then season. Mix well, increase the heat and add the stock. Once it boils, cover the pan, reduce the heat and simmer for about 30 minutes.

To serve, season with black pepper. Any leftovers will freeze well.

Nutrition Tips
Cabbage is high in fibre and contains powerful antioxidants, including polyphenols, which are thought to improve digestion, as well protect against cardiovascular diseases.

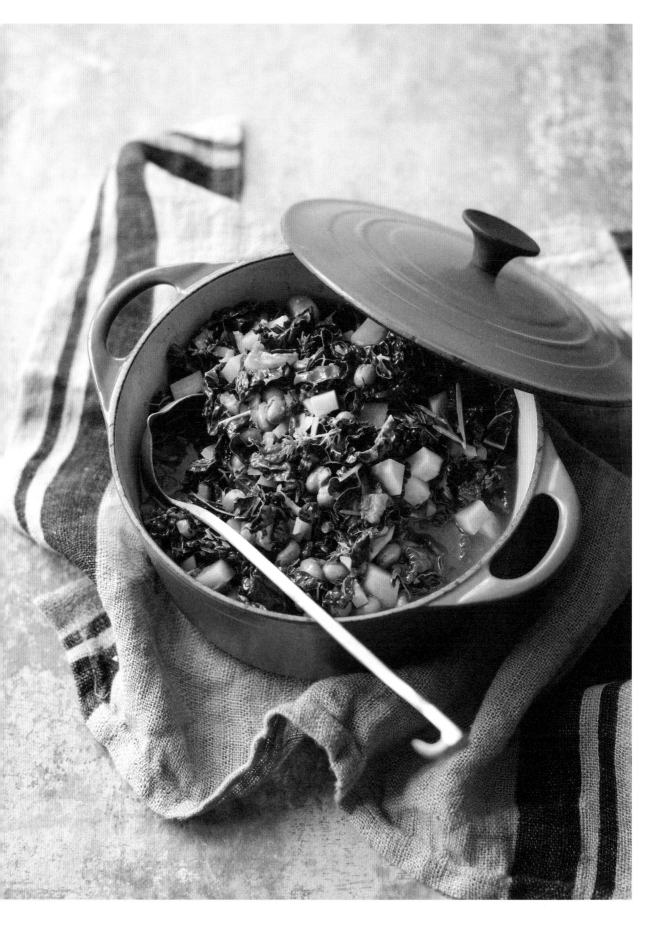

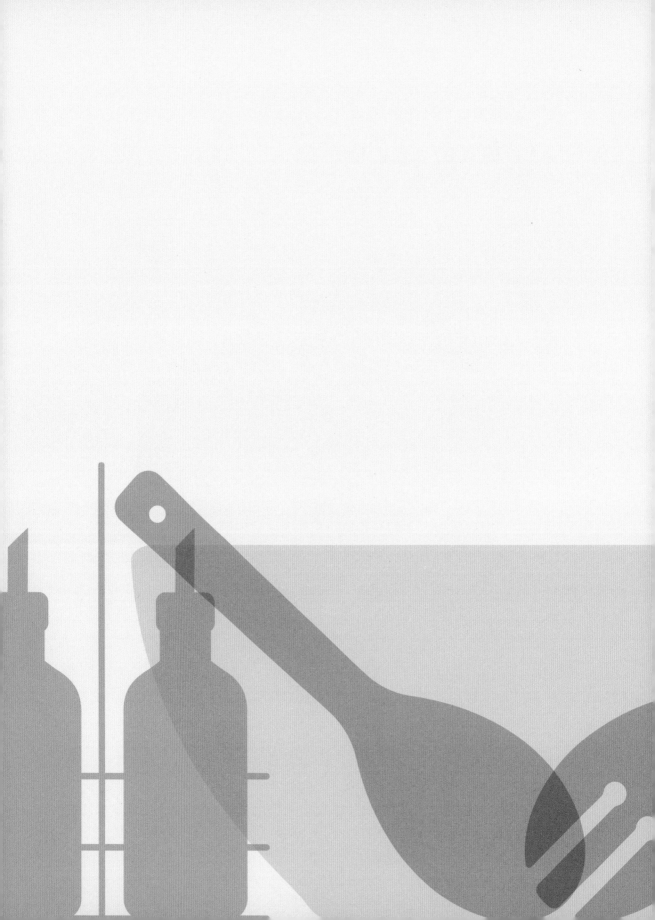

Salads, Sides & Dressings

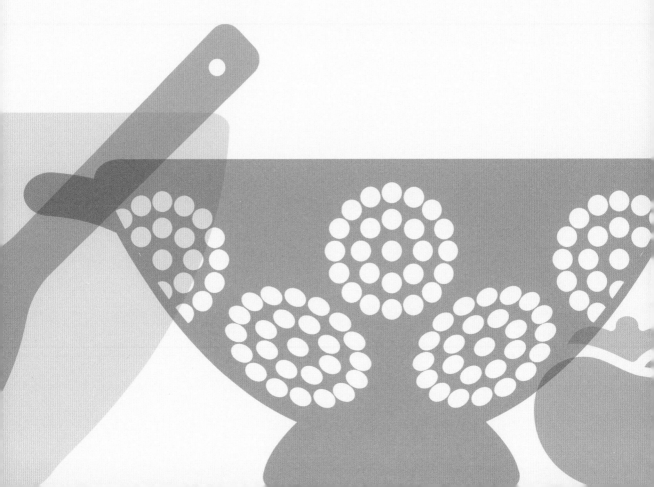

MED fat	MED sat	LOW sug	LOW salt	**ENERGY** 354kcals **PROTEIN** 42g | **FAT** 18g | **SATURATED FAT** 4.8g
18g	4.8g	0g	0.15g	**CARBOHYDRATE** 0g | **TOTAL SUGARS** 0g | **SALT** 0.15g | **SODIUM** 144mg | **FIBRE** 0g

Poached Chicken & Chicken Stock

Poached chicken may sound boring, but it is perfect to prepare ahead to make up a salad or packed lunch. To make homemade stock, you can use a cooked carcass leftover from a roast.

Poaching a whole chicken in advance will supply you with not only a batch of stock for the freezer, but also moist and tender chicken to make other meals. Plus it's cheaper, healthier and has less salt or additives than pre-cooked chicken from the deli.

Serves 4 / Makes 1 litre chicken stock

PREPARATION TIME: 15 minutes
COOKING TIME 1 hour 30 minutes

2 garlic cloves, crushed
selection of 'fridge' vegetables
  (e.g. celery, carrot)
1 onion, sliced
1 tablespoon sliced fresh ginger
  (optional)
1 small free-range chicken

Place all the ingredients except the chicken into a large pot with 1.5 litres of water and bring to the boil. Reduce the heat to a gentle simmer. Lower the chicken, breast-side down, into the simmering stock, fully submerged if possible. Poach the chicken gently for 1 hour. There should be no more than an occasional ripple breaking the surface; adjust the temperature, if necessary, to ensure the water does not boil. Keep an occasional eye on the pan so it doesn't boil dry.

You could do this in a slow cooker; just increase the cooking time for your type of cooker.

Remove the stockpot from the heat and, using tongs, gently remove the chicken from the stock. Place the chicken on a tray to drain and allow to cool.

Remove the skin, portion into breasts and legs and pull any meat from the carcass. Cover tightly and refrigerate if using later; it will keep in the fridge for up to 3 days.

Strain the stock and chill it so you can skim off the fat. Once skimmed, the stock is ready to use, or you can freeze it in portions to use for another dish.

Cook's Tip
Here are two ways to try with this poached chicken: Chicken Salad with Tomatoes, Olives and Capers (see page 63) or Chef's Chicken Salad with Quinoa (see page 64).

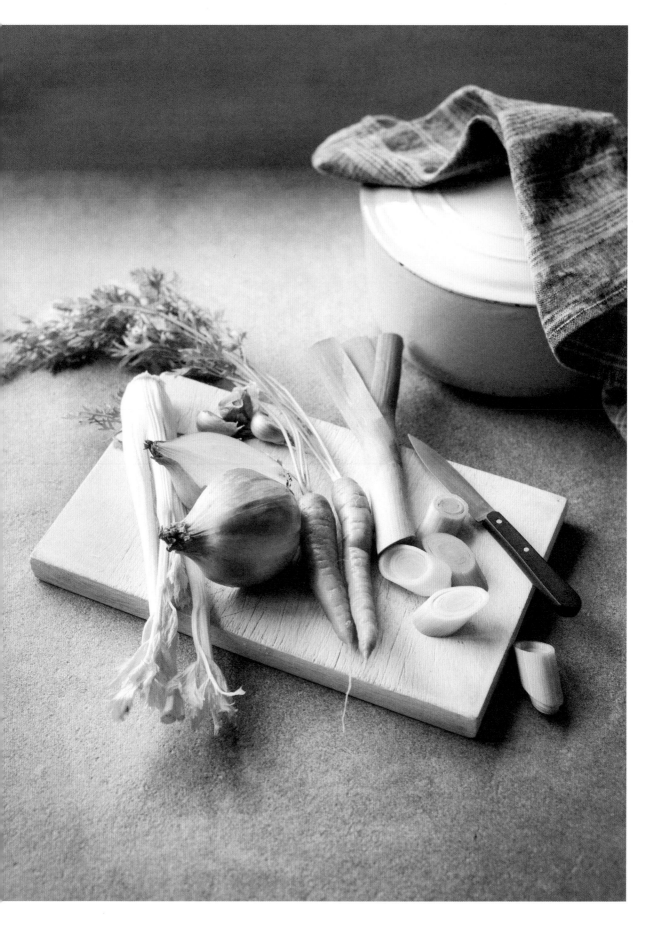

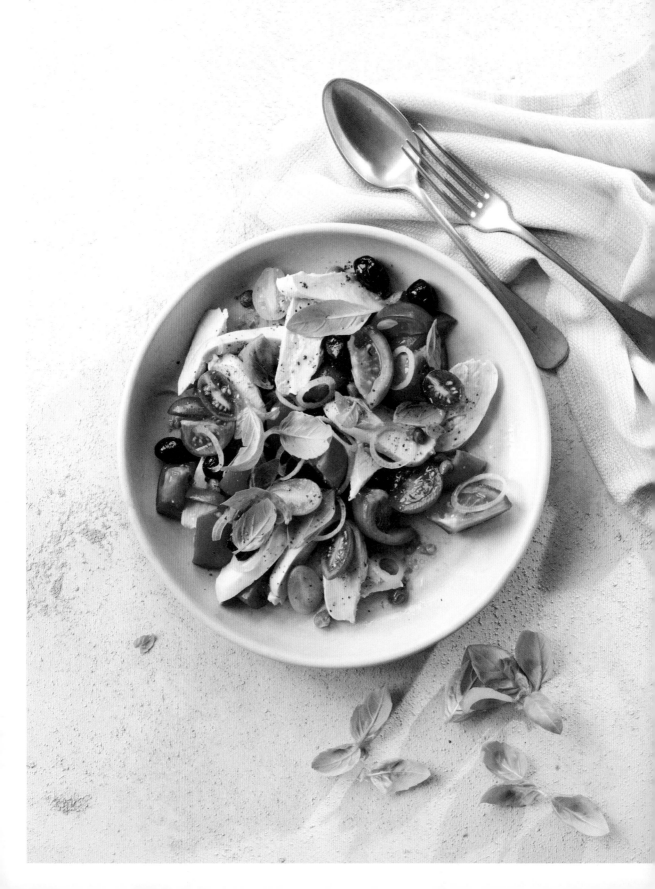

ENERGY 325kcals **PROTEIN** 39g | **FAT** 11g | **SATURATED FAT** 1.9g
CARBOHYDRATE 5.8g | **TOTAL SUGARS** 4.4g | **SALT** 1.3g | **SODIUM** 516mg | **FIBRE** 2.7g

Chicken Salad with Tomatoes, Olives and Capers

Sometimes simple can be best and with the capers, this is a punchy little salad. Use the most flavoursome kind of tomatoes you can find; it will make all the difference to the taste.

Serves 2

PREPARATION TIME: 10 minutes, plus marinating

1 small shallot, sliced into fine rings
250g ripe mixed tomatoes, cut into bite-size pieces
1 teaspoon capers
40g black olives, stoned
10 fresh basil leaves, torn or roughly chopped, plus extra to serve
2 teaspoons extra virgin olive oil
2 small chicken breasts (140g), poached, skinned and cooled (see page 60)
freshly ground black pepper

Mix the shallot, tomatoes, capers, olives and basil with the oil and a grind of black pepper. Slice the chicken and stir gently through the tomato mixture. Cover, chill and leave the flavours to marinate for up to an hour, if you can.

Serve the chicken salad with all the tomato juices and a few extra fresh basil leaves or mint.

Cook's Tip
If you want to dress this salad up a bit, then use different coloured tomatoes.

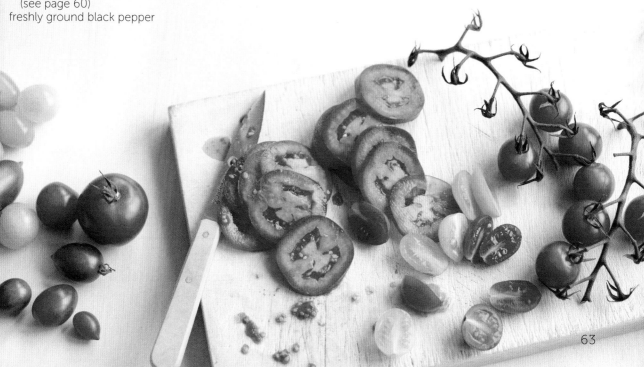

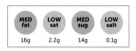

MED fat	LOW sat	MED sug	LOW salt
16g	2.2g	14g	0.1g

ENERGY 457kcals **PROTEIN** 33g | **FAT** 16g | **SATURATED FAT** 2.2g
CARBOHYDRATE 43g | **TOTAL SUGARS** 14g | **SALT** 0.1g | **SODIUM** 54mg | **FIBRE** 8.8g

Chef's Chicken Salad with Quinoa

This is a great salad to take on a picnic or, fingers crossed for the weather, a barbecue; keep it chilled until ready to eat. As the chef, you can chop and change the main ingredients: chicken or salmon, or make it vegetarian.

Serves 2

PREPARATION TIME: 15 minutes

1 tablespoon extra virgin olive oil
½ teaspoon Dijon mustard
juice of 1 small lime
100g quinoa, cooked and drained
¼ large fresh red chilli
2 spring onions, sliced diagonally
   (including the green part)
1 small red pepper, deseeded and
   finely chopped
2 tablespoons edamame beans or
   peas, cooked
20g dried sour cherries, cranberries
   or sultanas
a small handful of parsley or
   coriander, chopped, plus extra
   to serve
150g cooked chicken, thinly sliced
   or pulled from the legs of leftover
   poached or roasted chicken
   (see page 60)
spinach and watercress or micro
   salad leaves, to serve
freshly ground black pepper

Whisk together the oil, Dijon mustard and lime juice.

In a large bowl, fluff up the quinoa with a fork and mix in the rest of the ingredients, except the chicken, then add the mustard dressing. You can mix in the chicken together with the other ingredients, if you like, otherwise it looks nicer if you put the sliced chicken on top to serve.

Season well with black pepper and a few more herbs, then serve with the spinach and watercress or micro salad leaves.

Nutrition Tips
Parsley is a rich source of vitamin C.

Quinoa is one of the most nutrient-dense grains and a great source of protein because it contains all nine essential amino acids. Fibre can be beneficial to keep you fuller and more satisfied. Dietary fibre can be helpful to regulate the digestive system and can help you manage your diabetes.

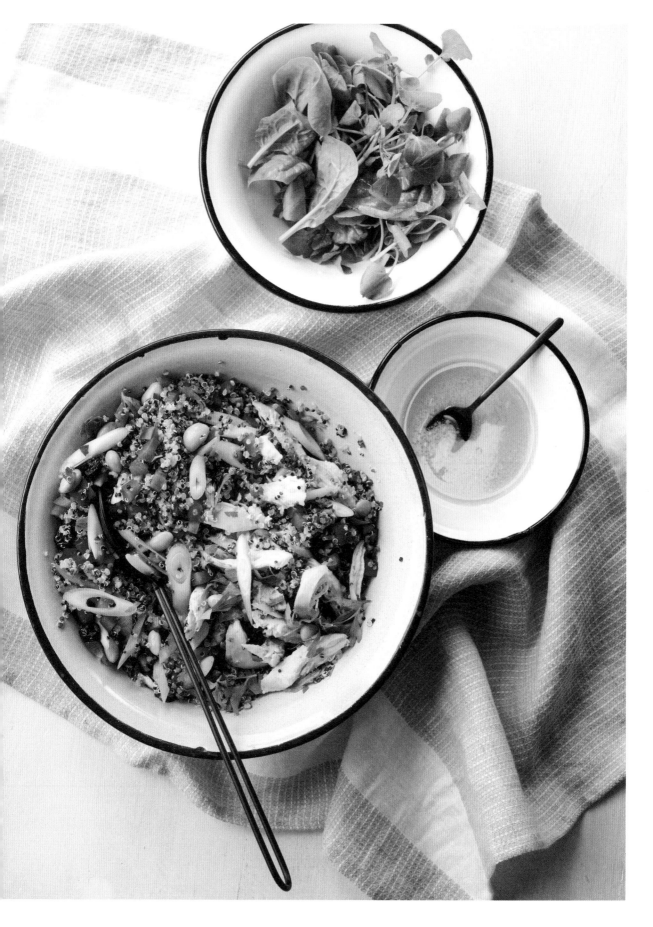

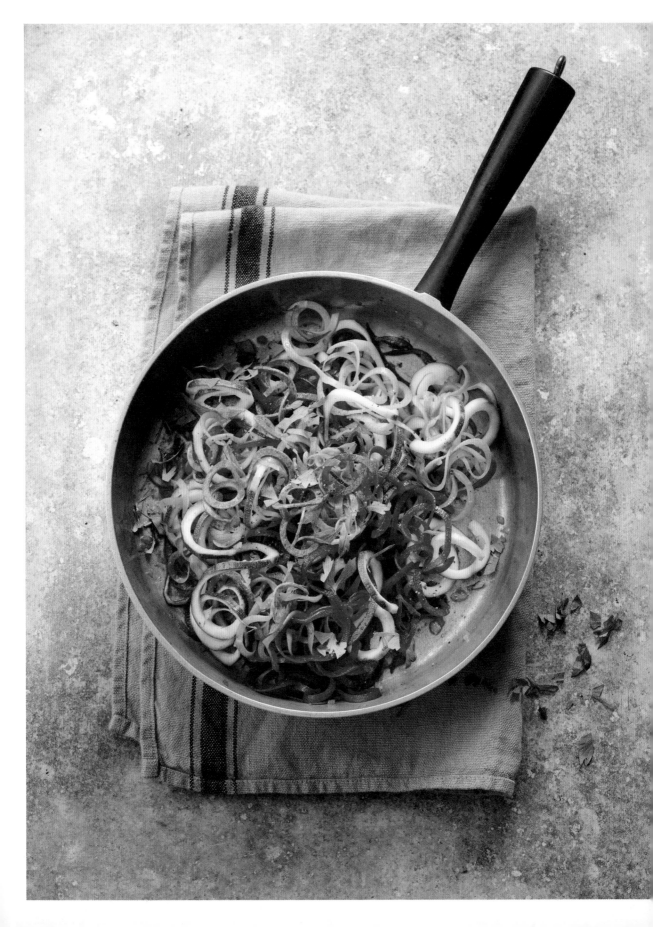

ENERGY 57kcals **PROTEIN** 3.7g | **FAT** 3.1g | **SATURATED FAT** 0.3g
CARBOHYDRATE 3.6g | **TOTAL SUGARS** 3.4g | **SALT** 0.1g | **SODIUM** 25mg | **FIBRE** 2.1g

Vegetable Noodles with Spicy Garlic Dressing

Some vegetables will happily lend themselves to make a delicious alternative for noodles and pasta. The vegetable noodles are also good to sauté for stir-fries, simmer briefly for soup or eat raw in salads. It helps if you have a spiraliser gadget with a special blade to turn any firm vegetable into strands. A rainbow of courgette, carrot, sweet potato and beetroot noodles are all delicious, lower calorie and lower carb, with more fibre than noodles or pasta. Here is a suggestion to use them for a side dish, dressed with a lightly spiced sauce.

Serves 2 as a side

PREPARATION TIME: 15 minutes
COOKING TIME: 10 minutes

FOR THE NOODLES
2 courgettes or a mixture of firm vegetables (e.g. 1 courgette and 1 carrot or 1 purple sweet potato)

FOR THE SAUCE
1 teaspoon rapeseed oil
1 shallot, finely chopped
2 garlic cloves, crushed
1–2 teaspoons Sriracha chilli sauce
juice of ½ lemon
1 tablespoon 0%-fat unsweetened Greek-style yogurt

TO SERVE
fresh parsley, chopped
freshly ground black pepper

Spiralise the vegetables if you have a spiraliser blade; alternatively, slice the ends off the vegetables, cut into long pieces and slice each thinly along the length. Then slice again into narrow strips, like noodles. You'll need about 300g prepared weight.

Cook the spiralised vegetables lightly: plunge into boiling water for 2–3 minutes and leave to drain well.

To make the sauce, heat a non-stick frying pan over a medium heat, add the oil and the shallot and cook for 3–4 minutes until softened. Add the garlic, 1 teaspoon of the chilli sauce, the lemon juice and 1 tablespoon of water, then heat for a minute or two until bubbling. Taste to see if you need the extra teaspoon of chilli sauce.

Add the vegetable 'noodles' to the hot pan, tossing them for couple of minutes until just coated with the sauce and hot through. Stir in the yogurt and remove from the heat.

Serve with cracked black pepper and parsley.

Cook's Tip
Sriracha is a hot and spicy chilli sauce; you don't need to add too much. If you like to prepare ahead, spiralised vegetable noodles will keep in a container in the fridge for 2–3 days and they freeze well. You can buy them already prepared, too.

LOW fat	LOW sat	LOW sug	LOW salt	**ENERGY** 21kcals	**PROTEIN** 2.1g	**FAT** 0.4g	**SATURATED FAT** 0g
0.4g	0g	2.1g	0.1g	**CARBOHYDRATE** 2.7g	**TOTAL SUGARS** 2.1g	**SALT** 0.1g	**SODIUM** 41mg	**FIBRE** 2.2g

Fennel Slaw Salad

GF

This is a colourful salad, which came from the idea of tweaking coleslaw to be a bit healthier. It will serve well with some grilled fish, or strips of steak and sweet potato wedges.

Serves 4 as a side

PREPARATION TIME: 15 minutes

¼ small red cabbage (75g)
1 small fennel bulb (125g), trimmed
2 spring onions, finely sliced
20g parsley, finely chopped
75g red chicory

FOR THE DRESSING
3 tablespoons (50g) 0%-fat
   unsweetened Greek-style yogurt
1 tablespoon lemon juice or apple
   cider vinegar
½ teaspoon Dijon mustard
pinch of chilli flakes (optional)
freshly ground black pepper

Finely shred the cabbage, removing any thick core stems. Slice the fennel finely, reserving any feathery, green tops to add with the parsley. Mix the prepared vegetables together in a large bowl and add the spring onions and the parsley.

Mix all of the ingredients for the dressing and toss with the salad in the bowl. Coat well and refrigerate for at least an hour to let the flavours soften into the salad ingredients.

When you are ready to serve, wash and separate the chicory bulb into leaves and then mix with the salad.

Cook's Tip

You could add a small apple, skin on, to naturally sweeten this salad: Quarter and core the apple, shred finely and add with the dressing ingredients. If you find the dressing is too sharp, add a tiny pinch of sweetener.

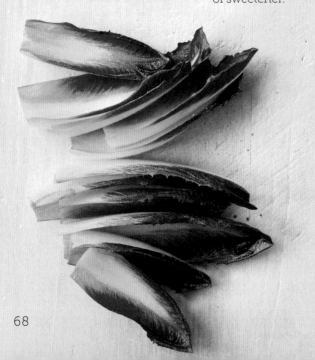

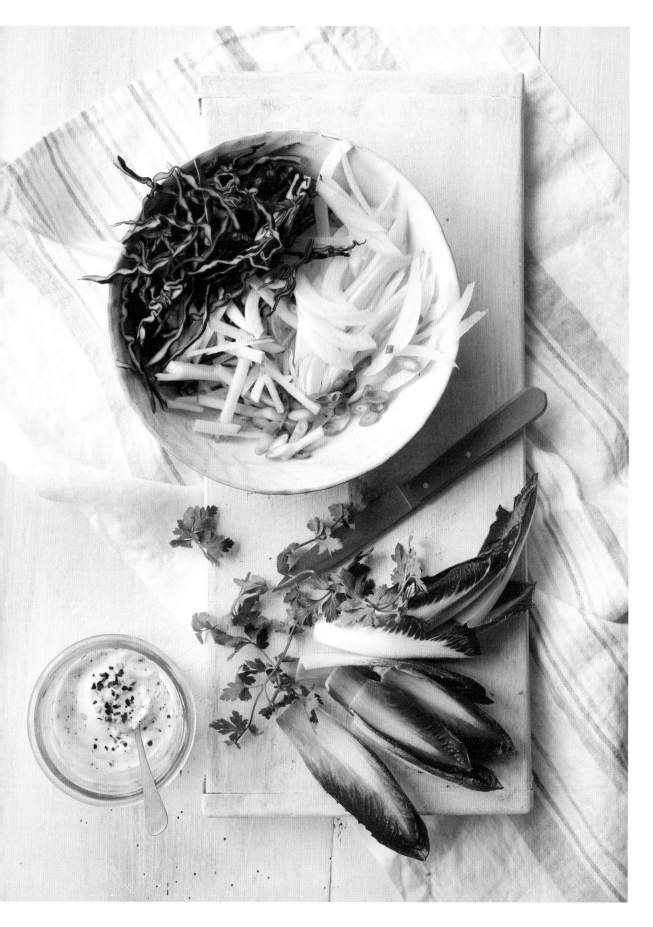

Nutrition Tip
Sweet potatoes have significantly more potassium, calcium and vitamin K than normal potatoes, plus they contain powerful antioxidant carotenes that can help promote healthy eyesight and good immune function.

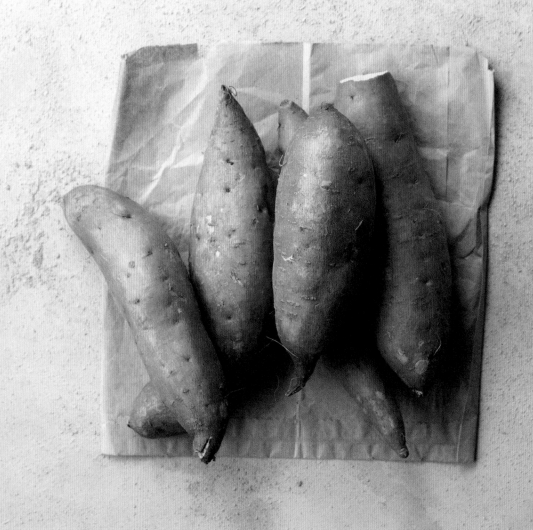

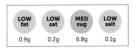

ENERGY 110kcals **PROTEIN** 1.4g | **FAT** 0.9g | **SATURATED FAT** 0.2g
CARBOHYDRATE 26g | **TOTAL SUGARS** 6.8g | **SALT** 0.1g | **SODIUM** 48mg | **FIBRE** 3.8g

Sweet Potato Fries

I've given the amount for one portion of oven-baked chips here, so you can easily scale up to how many you are serving. Smaller portions are the way to go and only cooking what you need each meal will also avoid food waste.

Serves 1

PREPARATION TIME: 5 minutes

COOKING TIME 25 minutes

1 small sweet potato (approx. 120g)
1-calorie vegetable oil cooking spray
½ teaspoon dried spice mix
 (optional: see tip)

Preheat the oven to 200°C/180°C/gas mark 6 and line a baking tray with greaseproof paper.

Scrub the sweet potato skin with water to clean and then dry. Slice into thick-cut fries, leaving the skin on.

Place in a single layer on the baking tray and spray lightly with the vegetable oil. Sprinkle over an even coating of spice seasoning, if using. Bake in the oven for about 25 minutes.

These are best served straight away – and so much better than the shop-bought ones.

Cook's Tip
For the spice mix, I like a Spanish bravas mix of spicy smoked paprika and dried oregano.

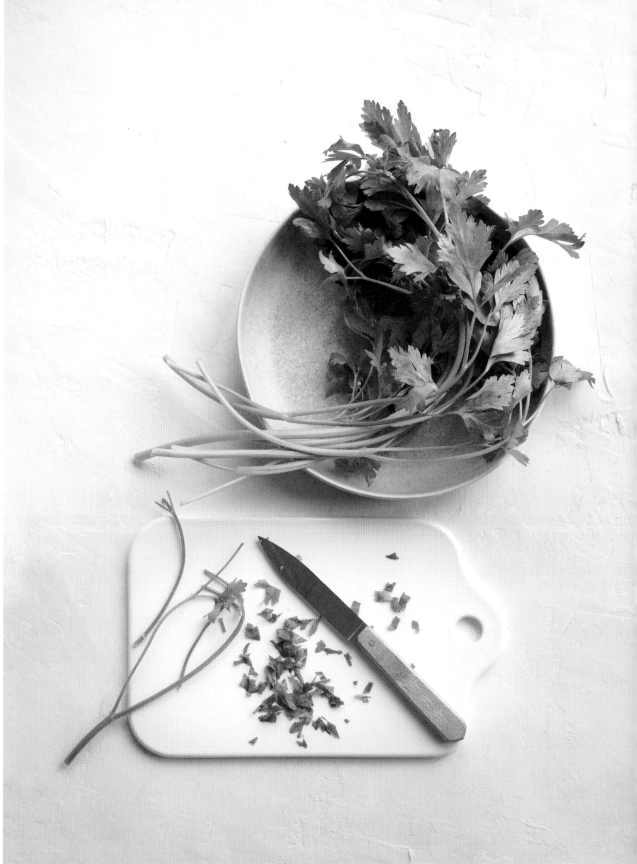

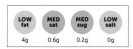

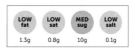

ENERGY 41kcals **PROTEIN** 0.4g | **FAT** 4g
SATURATED FAT 0.6g | **CARBOHYDRATE** 0.9g
TOTAL SUGARS 0.2g | **SALT** 0g | **SODIUM** 3mg | **FIBRE** 1g

ENERGY 73kcals **PROTEIN** 6.2g | **FAT** 1.3g
SATURATED FAT 0.8g | **CARBOHYDRATE** 10g
TOTAL SUGARS 10g | **SALT** 0.1g | **SODIUM** 81mg | **FIBRE** 0.4g

Chimichurri Herb Dressing

This version of the South American herb dressing is made with parsley, oregano and chilli and adds a slightly sharp distinction for salads, grilled meats or vegetables. You can use it as a marinade, too.

Serves 4

PREPARATION TIME: 5 minutes

2 tablespoons finely chopped parsley
2 tablespoons finely chopped oregano or marjoram
1 teaspoon red wine vinegar
1 teaspoon lemon juice
1 small garlic clove, crushed
1 tablespoon olive oil
tiny pinch of chilli flakes

Combine all the ingredients in a small bowl with 1 tablespoon of water and then leave to sit and mingle the flavours for a while: it's also good to make the day before.

Cook's Tips

For snacking, take a Little Gem lettuce and separate the leaves into 'cups' to eat with a spoonful of this chimichurri dressing.

Summer Herb Yogurt

The simplest of snacks.

Serves 4

PREPARATION TIME: 5 minutes

a handful of fresh herbs, chopped (such as dill, parsley, mint and basil)
1 small garlic clove, crushed
500g pot low-fat unsweetened live yogurt

Fold the herbs and garlic into the live yogurt. Add some crisp red pepper on the side; or try roasting some fingers of beetroot to accompany.

Nutrition Tip

Garlic is an excellent source of manganese and vitamin B6. It also contains compounds that can help to reduce blood pressure.

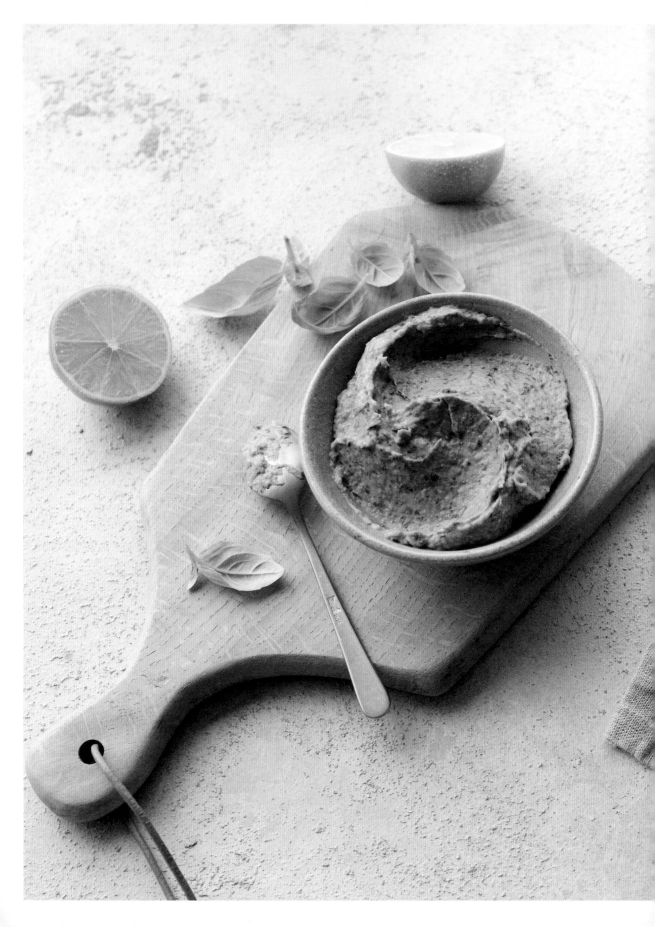

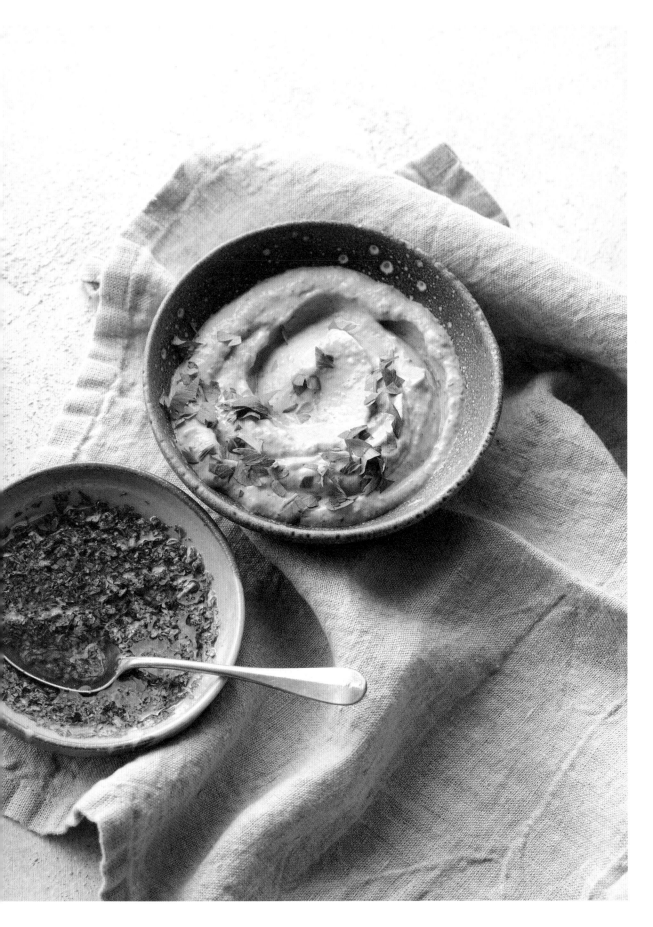

Two Green Vegan Dressings

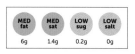

MED fat	MED sat	LOW sug	LOW salt
6g	1.4g	0.2g	0g

ENERGY 60kcals **PROTEIN** 0.7g | **FAT** 6g | **SATURATED FAT** 1.4g
CARBOHYDRATE 0.8g | **TOTAL SUGARS** 0.2g | **SALT** 0g | **SODIUM** 1.5mg | **FIBRE** 3g

Avocado & Herb Dressing

The natural creaminess of the avocado mixed with fresh herbs and a tang of vinegar or lime makes this a great match for vegetables and salads. Use it as a dip or spread for toast with an egg, or use in sandwiches.

Serves 4

PREPARATION TIME: 5 minutes

a small handful of fresh basil leaves, chopped
a small handful of fresh coriander leaves, stalks removed and leaves chopped
a small sliver of garlic, chopped
flesh of 1 small, ripe avocado
½ teaspoon lime juice or apple cider vinegar

Garlic can overpower the flavour of this dip if you add too much, and similarly, a heavy spoon of the citrus juice or vinegar can spoil the result: start with less and you can always taste and add more.

Put the herbs and garlic in a small blender and pulse to a rough paste. Add the avocado and drops of the lime juice or vinegar and pulse until combined to a smooth 'dip'. Some finely sliced spring onions would be nice to serve with this.

Cook's Tip
Sometimes I simplify this one and just blend half an avocado with a roasted red pepper and a squeeze of lime juice, instead of the herbs.

Nutrition Tip
Avocados are naturally rich in heart-healthy monounsaturated fats, useful fibre and vitamin E.

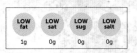

ENERGY 25kcals **PROTEIN** 2.8g | **FAT** 1g | **SATURATED FAT** 0g

CARBOHYDRATE 1g | **TOTAL SUGARS** 0g | **SALT** 0g | **SODIUM** 2mg | **FIBRE** 0g

Herb & Tofu Green Dressing

Ve

GF

If you haven't tried tofu yet, give it a go. It's a really versatile ingredient made from soya beans: a good source of vegetarian protein, calcium and minerals. This dressing calls for 'silken' smooth, soft tofu, not the standard firm block of tofu. Silken tofu will transform into a creamy, thick dressing: a healthier swap for mayo dressings. This herby drizzle is great for a salad, on vegetables or as a burger sauce (see page 140).

Serves 4

PREPARATION TIME: 5 minutes

150g silken tofu
a small handful of fresh parsley, stalks removed and leaves chopped
a small handful of fresh basil leaves, chopped
a small sliver of garlic, chopped

Combine the ingredients in a small blender and blitz until smooth. When you see how thick the dressing is, add up to 1 tablespoon of water if you want a thinner drizzle.

Transfer to a clean container, such as a jar, and store in the fridge for up to 2 days. If you have some spare tofu, store it, covered in water, in a small container in the fridge.

Cook's Tip

As an alternative to the herbs, you can just flavour the soft tofu with a teaspoon each of Dijon mustard and lemon juice and use as a creamy 'mayo'.

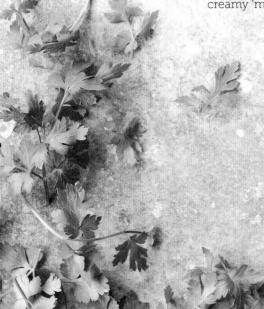

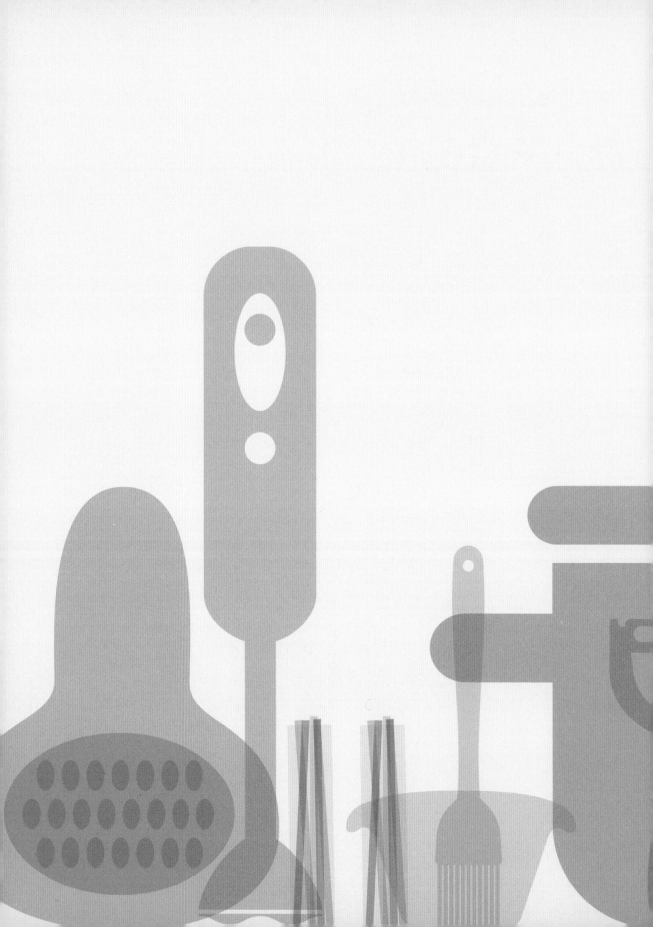

Vegetarian & Vegan

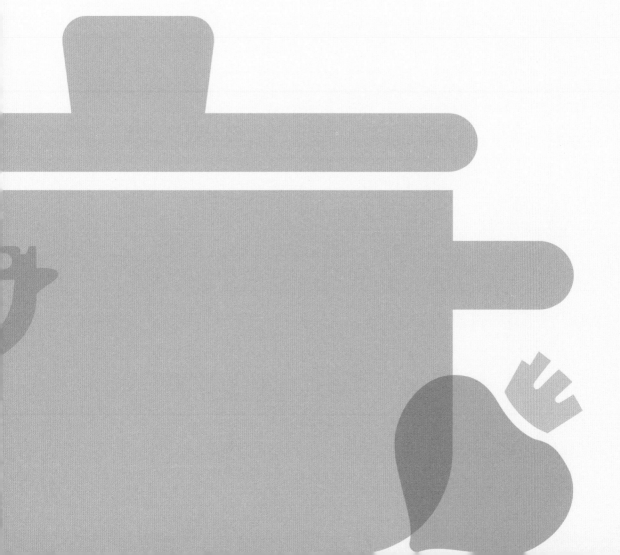

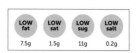

ENERGY 279kcals **PROTEIN** 15g | **FAT** 7.5g | **SATURATED FAT** 1.5g
CARBOHYDRATE 40g | **TOTAL SUGARS** 11g | **SALT** 0.2g | **SODIUM** 119mg | **FIBRE** 13g

Vegetable Scramble

I cook this dish a couple of ways. It's a great way to use up leftover cooked vegetables, from a Sunday roast for instance, or I cook it with fish or meat; the ideas are endless. Whichever way I'm cooking this dish, I sometimes pop the pan into a very hot oven to warm through and get a little colour; this is a great trick if you are using little or no oil. If you are following this route, then preheat the oven to 230°C/210°C/gas mark 8. Here I use a selection of cooked vegetables, but any will do really; sometimes I even use a pack of mixed frozen veg or certain canned varieties.

Serves 2

PREPARATION TIME: 10 minutes
COOKING TIME: 15 minutes

1 teaspoon rapeseed oil
200g cooked potatoes, chopped
200g cooked cauliflower, cut into
   small florets
200g cooked carrots, chopped
200g cooked green beans
1 egg
1 egg white
100g frozen peas, defrosted
freshly ground black pepper

Heat the oil in a non-stick large frying pan. Add all of the vegetables apart from the peas. Cook over a high heat for about 6–8 minutes, until they take on a little colour and warm through.

Break up the whole egg and egg white and, with the pan still over the heat, pour over the egg and stir quickly through the vegetables so that it coagulates and coats the vegetables well. Add the peas and a little salt and pepper and serve straight away.

Nutrition Tip
Peas have been part of the human diet for hundreds of years and are consumed all over the world. Plus they are low in calories and high in protein.

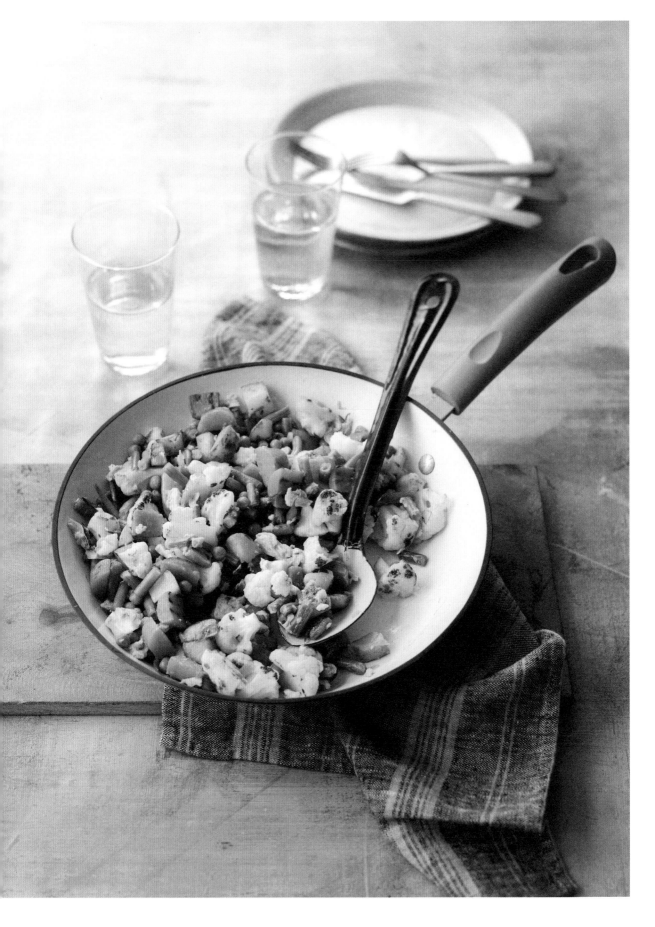

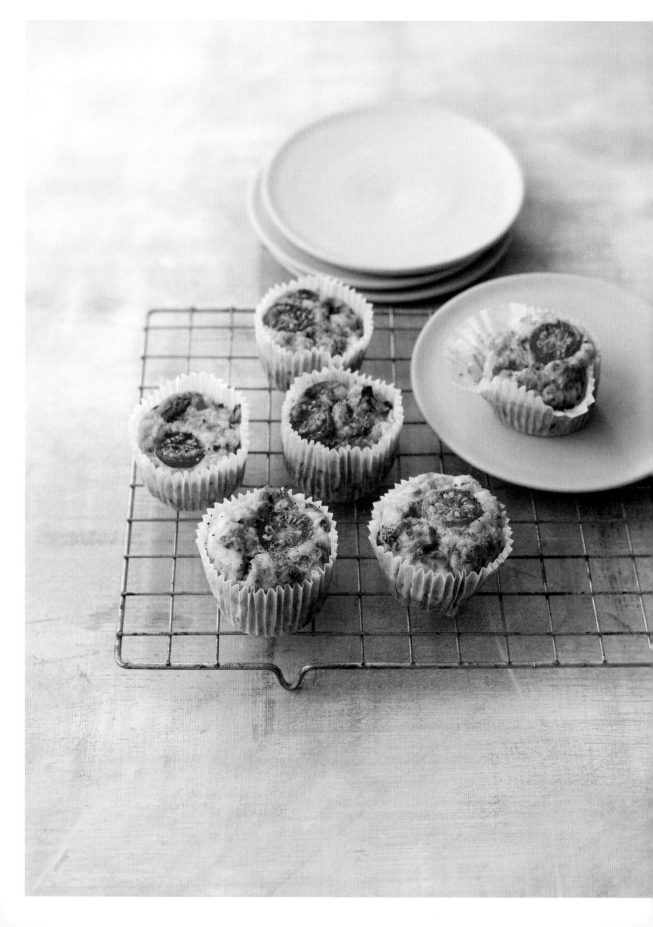

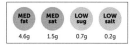

ENERGY 73kcals **PROTEIN** 7.2g | **FAT** 4.6g | **SATURATED FAT** 1.5g
CARBOHYDRATE 0.7g | **TOTAL SUGARS** 0.7g | **SALT** 0.2g | **SODIUM** 97mg | **FIBRE** 0.3g

MED fat	MED sat	LOW sug	LOW salt
4.6g	1.5g	0.7g	0.2g

Tortilla Muffins

This neat recipe is great for using up leftover bits of cooked veg, plus combining them with eggs give the dish a nutritious contribution of protein, vitamins and minerals.

Makes 6

PREPARATION TIME: 15 minutes
COOKING TIME: 20 minutes

4 sprays 1-calorie sunflower oil
   cooking spray
1 banana shallot, finely chopped
30g chopped pepper
4 eggs
1 tablespoon 0%-fat unsweetened
   Greek-style yogurt (see tip)
a few basil leaves, chopped, or
   a pinch of dried herbs
freshly ground black pepper

FOR THE TOPPING
30g reduced-fat Cheddar, grated
3 cherry tomatoes, halved

Preheat the oven to 200°C/180°C fan/gas mark 6 and line a muffin tin with six cases. The cooked egg mixture tends to stick to the cases, so ideally use a non-stick silicone mould tray, so the contents pop out easily and no oil is needed.

Heat the cooking spray in a small pan and fry the shallot and pepper until softened, about 5–8 minutes. At this point you could include any little extra bits like sautéed mushrooms or a handful of chopped spinach leaves, to wilt at the end.

Beat the eggs with the yogurt, herbs and seasoning in a small jug, add the cooked vegetables and mix all together. Pour the egg mixture into the six cups, half-filling each one. Sprinkle with cheese, press half a cherry tomato on top and bake for about 15–20 minutes until set.

Nutrition Tip
Though these recipes use low-fat dairy, try using other unsweetened alternatives such as small amounts of full-fat dairy, which contains some beneficial fats, live yogurt or even cottage cheese.

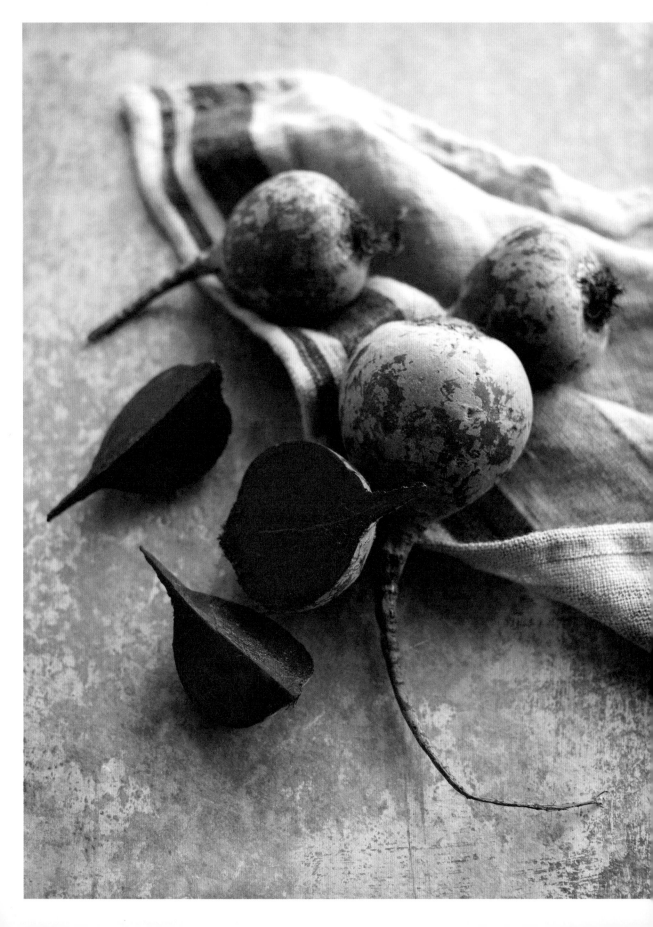

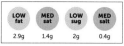
Beetroot & Feta Falafels

I love these moreish and pleasingly pink falafels; the earthy flavour of beetroot is softened by the cheese and just a hint of mint and herb. They are delicious hot or cold, as a snack or for a casual lunch with some salad and cherry tomatoes. This recipe makes ten because if you are going to the effort of making them, you may as well make extra to freeze for instant falafel next time. Or you can easily just halve everything here.

Makes 10

PREPARATION TIME: 15 minutes
COOKING TIME: 20 minutes

200g beetroot, cooked and cubed
75g feta, cubed
2 eggs
100g wholemeal breadcrumbs
30g spring onions, chopped
1 tablespoon finely chopped fresh
    mint leaves
½ teaspoon finely chopped
    rosemary leaves
1 small garlic clove, crushed
    or grated
freshly ground black pepper

Preheat the oven to 180°C/160°C fan/gas mark 4. Line a baking tray with greaseproof paper.

Put the cubes of beetroot into a food-processor or blender and pulse until you have small chunks. You want the raw mixture to be quite dry, which depends on the type of beetroot you are using: if it's fresh, roasted beetroot then it will be dry, otherwise, remove the lid and pour away any excess liquid if it looks runny before you add the rest of the ingredients.

Add all the remaining ingredients to the food-processor and blend until evenly just mixed.

Using a large tablespoon, scoop the soft mixture into ten slightly flattened balls and drop onto the baking tray. Bake in the oven for about 20 minutes, until lightly firm and cooked through.

Cook's Tip

Serve one as a snack – no need to add pitta bread. Or, for a light lunch: split and warm a 20g mini pitta bread. Stuff with one falafel, 15g chopped cucumber, some rocket salad or fennel slaw (see page 68) and a teaspoon of unsweetened Greek-style yogurt. Add slices of chilli to make it spicy.

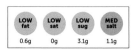

ENERGY 57kcals **PROTEIN** 2.4g | **FAT** 0.6g | **SATURATED FAT** 0g
CARBOHYDRATE 11g | **TOTAL SUGARS** 3.1g | **SALT** 1.1g | **SODIUM** 425mg | **FIBRE** 2.6g

Vegetable Spring Rolls

If using gluten-free soy sauce

When I filmed in Mekong Delta, spring rolls were on every boat, street and food vendor's stall. Most had very little or no meat at all, relying instead on great flavours. Here is a vegetable version with no cooking at all. If you eat meat, you could add a little cooked chicken breast, a few prawns or a little tuna if you wanted to. Or you could steam the rolls for a hot version.

Serves 4

PREPARATION TIME: 35–40 minutes

FOR THE DRESSING
1 teaspoon fresh red chilli, very finely chopped
1 garlic clove, crushed
2 teaspoons reduced-salt soy sauce
2 tablespoons rice wine vinegar
4 tablespoons chopped Thai or any fresh basil
4 tablespoons chopped fresh mint
4 tablespoons chopped fresh coriander
freshly ground black pepper

FOR THE ROLLS
1 medium carrot, peeled and cut into very fine strips
6 spring onions, cut into very fine strips
½ small cucumber, cut into very fine strips
1 pak choi, cut into very fine strips
16 dried rice paper wrappers

FOR THE DIPPING SAUCE
4 tablespoons rice wine vinegar
1 teaspoon soy sauce
1 small red chilli, finely chopped
2 tablespoons chopped coriander
1 teaspoon granulated sweetener
juice of 1 lime

Place all the ingredients for the dressing into a bowl and mix well. Add the vegetables and really mix well.

Make the dipping sauce by mixing all the ingredients in a small bowl.

Lightly moisten the rice paper sheets with a pastry brush and a little water until they are pliable but not soggy. Place a little of the dressed vegetables into the centre of the wrapper and fold in the sides. Roll up from the bottom and seal well. Repeat with the other 15 wrappers.

Serve with the dipping sauce as a nice starter, snack or light lunch.

Nutrition Tips
Spring onions are a good source of dietary fibre as well as vitamins C, A and B6.

Cucumbers are low in calories but contain high amounts of soluble fibre.

Pak choi belongs to the same cruciferous family as kale and cauliflower. Also low in calories, it's a good source of vitamins C and E and beta-carotene.

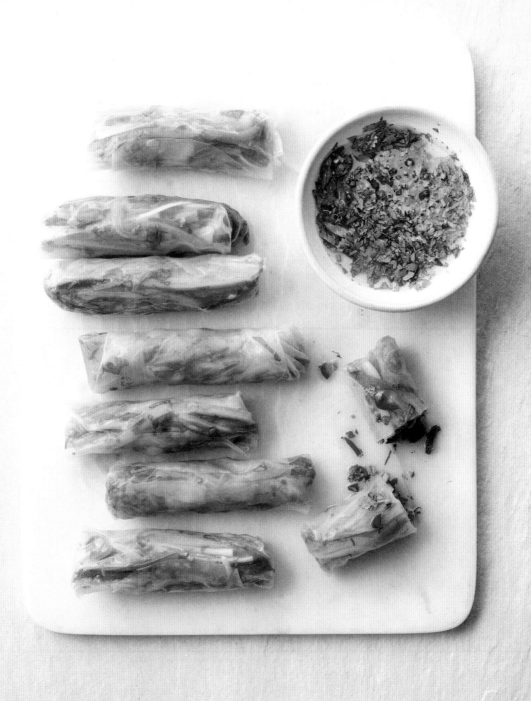

Tomato & Feta Balls

While on holiday in Greece, I ate something similar to these tomato snacks. I was fond of the similar courgette version they had, too, but both were fried and laden with oil. A good way to lower the fat in fried food is to bake it instead. The gram flour is made from chickpeas and adds some protein, too.

Makes 4

PREPARATION TIME: 10 minutes
COOKING TIME: 20 minutes

4 sprays 1-calorie olive oil cooking spray
7 cherry tomatoes (100g), chopped
1 teaspoon tomato purée
2 spring onions, chopped (including the green parts)
20g feta, chopped
a small handful of fresh mint, chopped
¼ teaspoon dried oregano
4 tablespoons gram (chickpea) flour

Preheat the oven to 200°C/180°C fan/gas mark 6. Line a baking tray with a sheet of non-stick baking paper and spray the paper lightly with the cooking spray.

Put the tomatoes, purée, spring onions, feta, mint and oregano into a food-processor (or use a stick blender) and process to mush them together briefly; it shouldn't be too smooth. Scrape the mixture out into a small bowl and add the gram flour. Stir until it makes a thick and sticky paste.

Form the mixture into four balls and place on the baking sheet. Bake for 10 minutes and then turn them over to cook on the other side for another 10 minutes until firm. The ones I had in Greece were oval in shape; although it doesn't matter much, they are soft when they are just cooked so you can push the edges into a neater shape, if you prefer.

Cook's Tip
Enjoy with a spoon of tzatziki; mix together some unsweetened Greek-style yogurt, garlic, lemon juice and chopped cucumber to taste.

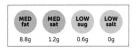

MED fat	MED sat	LOW sug	LOW salt
8.8g	1.2g	0.6g	0g

ENERGY 156kcals **PROTEIN** 5.7g | **FAT** 8.8g | **SATURATED FAT** 1.2g
CARBOHYDRATE 14g | **TOTAL SUGARS** 0.6g | **SALT** 0g | **SODIUM** 0mg | **FIBRE** 2g

Savoury Socca Pancakes

This is such a simple recipe for savoury pancakes, which can make a great lunch or supper snack. Serve it flat, like a pizza, topped with anything that takes your fancy.

The recipe originates from Nice in France as socca (or farinata in Italy) and is a kind of flatbread made from chickpea flour and very little else. Chickpea flour is surprisingly useful, vegan friendly and gluten-free.

Makes 4 × 15cm pancakes

PREPARATION TIME: 5 minutes
COOKING TIME: 20 minutes

2 tablespoons extra virgin olive oil
125ml sparkling water
100g gram (chickpea) flour
½ teaspoon dried mixed herbs
1-calorie vegetable oil cooking
   spray, for frying
freshly ground black pepper

Combine the olive oil with the sparkling water and whisk into the gram flour until smooth. You don't have to use sparkling water, but I think it makes the batter slightly lighter. Add some herbs to make it more interesting: I like an Italian mix of oregano, marjoram, rosemary and thyme, but you can add anything such as spices and garlic. Season with black pepper.

Cook one pancake at a time, using a small non-stick frying pan with a heavy base. A good solid pan will need less oil to cook. Heat your pan over a high heat and add a couple of sprays of oil. Add a quarter of the batter to the pan and swirl it into a pancake shape. Allow to cook for about 2 minutes, until it is drying out on the surface and set around the edges – reduce the heat if it browns too quickly. Carefully lift up the pancake and flip it over to cook for another 2 minutes or so until golden. Remove and set aside to keep warm. Repeat with the rest of the batter.

Best eaten warm straight away, but leftovers can be stored in the fridge for up to 2 days and then warmed up.

Cook's Tip
Add an egg, fried in the same pan after you've made the pancakes, and spread the socca base with an infinite variety of savoury toppings; try the red pepper pesto from my recipe for Roasted Red Pepper & Sardines on Toast (see page 27) with some salad.

Nutrition Tip
Aubergines, like tomatoes, potatoes and peppers, belong to the nightshade family. They are high in fibre and low in fat. They also are rich in antioxidants, in particular nasunin, which gives their skin its purple colour, and may protect the lipids in brain cell membranes.

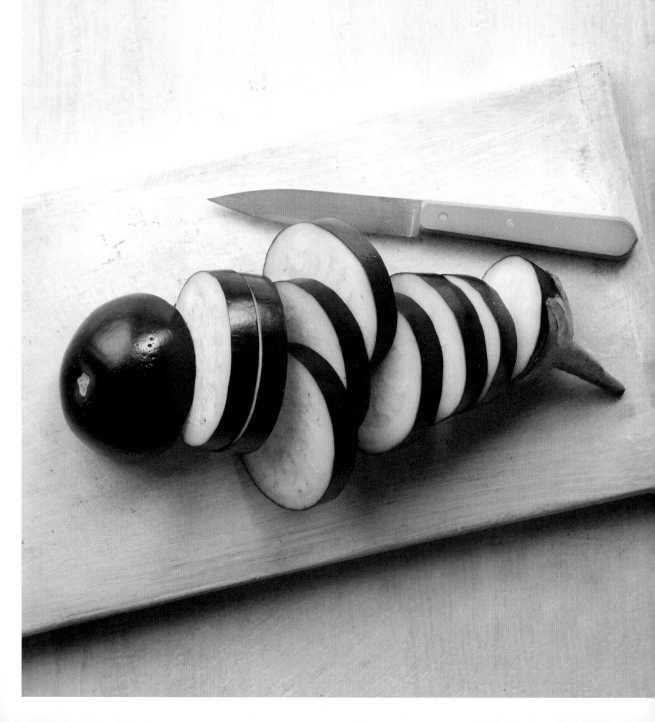

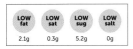

ENERGY 114kcals **PROTEIN** 7g | **FAT** 2.1g | **SATURATED FAT** 0.3g

CARBOHYDRATE 17g | **TOTAL SUGARS** 5.2g | **SALT** 0g | **SODIUM** 18mg | **FIBRE** 7.8g

Aubergine & Bean Burgers

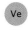

Aubergines can absorb a lot of oil when you fry them: a tip to avoid this is to pre-cook them slightly in the microwave first. Plus this softens them, which makes cooking much quicker, too.

Serves 4

PREPARATION TIME: 20 minutes, plus 30 minutes chilling
COOKING TIME: 25 minutes

1 small aubergine
1 teaspoon rapeseed oil
1 small red onion, finely chopped
1 small garlic clove, crushed
1 teaspoon ground cumin
1 teaspoon hot smoked paprika
   (or less spicy, to taste)
1 teaspoon wine vinegar
½ tablespoon tomato purée
120g can mixed beans, drained well
   and rinsed
70g cooked sweet potato, mashed
1 tablespoon gram (chickpea) flour
   (optional)
1-calorie vegetable oil cooking
   spray
freshly ground black pepper

First soften the aubergine in the microwave: prick the skin all over (otherwise it will pop), put the whole vegetable onto a microwaveable plate and heat on full power for 2–3 minutes. It should be quite soft and will be very hot to touch; remove carefully and leave to cool slightly.

Heat the oil in a large, non-stick pan over a medium heat. Add the onion and sauté for 5 minutes to soften. Chop the aubergine into very small pieces. (If you do this just before adding it to a hot pan, it will discolour less.)

Increase the heat a little, then stir-fry the aubergines with the onions for another 5 minutes. Then mix in the garlic, spices, vinegar and tomato purée; stir-fry for about 5 minutes more to finish cooking the aubergine, then season with black pepper.

Next roughly mash the mixed beans with the sweet potato; it doesn't have to be smooth. Tip the cooked vegetables into the bean mash and squidge the mixture until it all comes together. If the mixture is very soft, add the gram flour. Divide into four patties; they should be firm enough to hold their shape (if not, add more gram flour). Chill them for 30 minutes to firm before cooking.

To cook, heat a non-stick pan over a medium heat, spritz with oil and cook for about 4 minutes on each side.

Cook's Tip
Check out the Blueprint Burgers on page 140 for serving ideas.

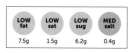

ENERGY 262kcals **PROTEIN** 17g | **FAT** 7.5g | **SATURATED FAT** 1.5g
CARBOHYDRATE 32g | **TOTAL SUGARS** 6.2g | **SALT** 0.4g | **SODIUM** 152mg | **FIBRE** 6.3g

Quinoa Chinese Leaf Mushroom Bowl with Poached Eggs

If using gluten-free stock cube

The mix of raw and cooked ingredients in this light lunch, or even breakfast dish, gives a nice texture and colour to the finished dish, as well as providing a good source of essential nutrients to contribute to a healthy diet. The Chinese leaves (or cabbage) have a mildly sweet flavour and crisp texture as well as containing useful vitamins and minerals, which may help to keep blood pressure within a healthy range.

Serves 4

PREPARATION TIME: 30 minutes
COOKING TIME: 20 minutes

200g quinoa, rinsed well
600ml boiling water
10g reduced-salt vegetable stock cube
2 garlic cloves, finely chopped
1 tablespoon finely grated fresh ginger
450g finely sliced button mushrooms
200g Chinese leaves, finely sliced
8 spring onions, sliced
1 medium carrot, peeled and very finely sliced into thin strips
4 poached eggs (see Cook's Tip)
freshly ground black pepper

Place the quinoa, water, stock cube, garlic, ginger and mushrooms into a saucepan, bring to the boil and add a little ground pepper. Stir well, reduce the heat and gently simmer for roughly 15 minutes.

Once the quinoa is cooked (all the stock should have been just about absorbed), remove the pan from the stove. Add the Chinese leaves, cover with a tight-fitting lid and leave for 15 minutes to soften.

Carefully fold the softened leaves into the quinoa, along with the spring onions. Spoon into a deep bowl, add the raw carrot and really mix well. Spoon into four bowls and top each one with the lightly poached eggs.

Cook's Tip

If you are poaching eggs, make sure the water is simmering and not boiling. Add a small dash of vinegar to the water. For the best results, use really fresh eggs: crack each egg into a ramekin dish so that you can easily tip it into the water. Stir the simmering water, making a little whirlpool in the pan and then gently tip the egg into the centre to poach. It will take about 5 minutes, depending on how cold the egg is to start with. Use a slotted spoon to remove the egg from the water and drain on kitchen paper.

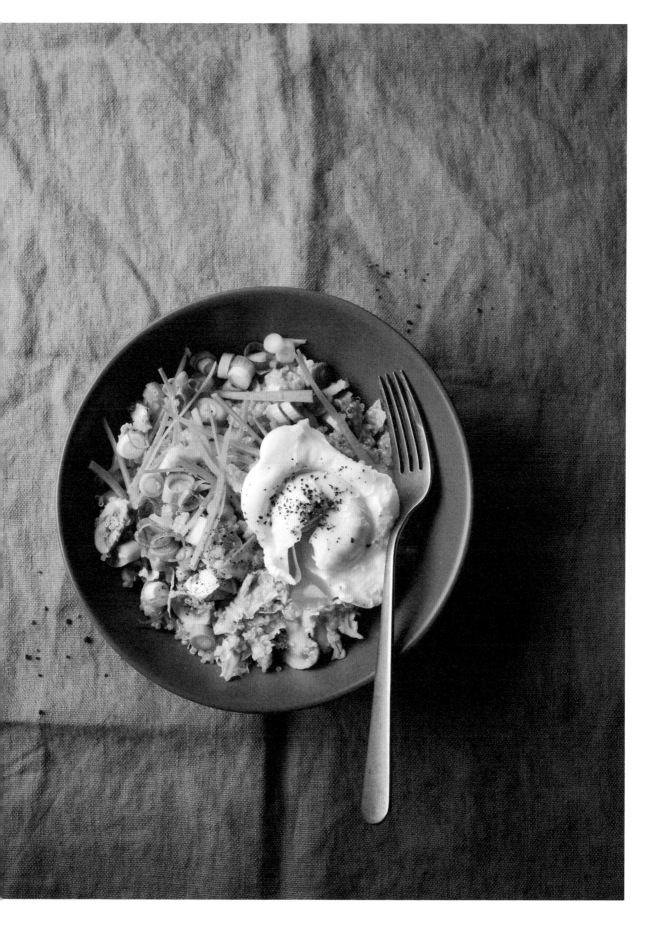

Nutrition Tip
Cauliflower is low in calories and a good source of vitamins C, K and B6, folate, pantothenic acid, choline, fibre, omega-3 fatty acids, manganese, phosphorus and biotin. It also contains vitamins B1 and B2, niacin and magnesium.

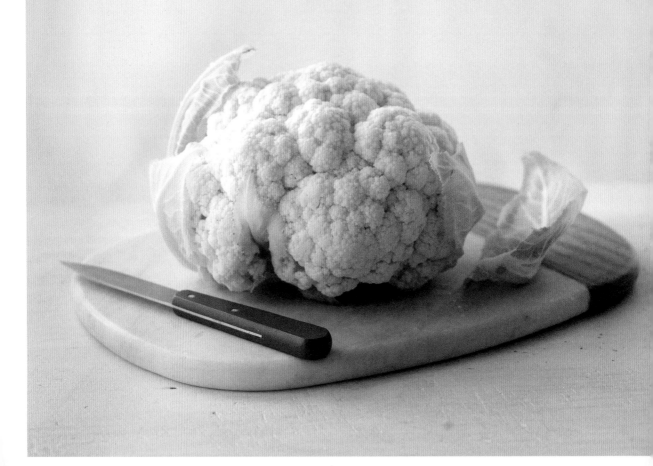

ENERGY 74kcals **PROTEIN** 5.5g | **FAT** 1.7g | **SATURATED FAT** 0.3g
CARBOHYDRATE 11g | **TOTAL SUGARS** 6g | **SALT** 0g | **SODIUM** 15mg | **FIBRE** 5g

Roasted Cauliflower Steaks

Oven-roasted, thick slices of cauliflower with a simple seasoning. Serve this as a veggie main with some mashed cannellini beans, or as a side vegetable instead of potatoes. Whole spices release great flavours but if you prefer not to bash the seeds, use ground spices.

Serves 4

PREPARATION TIME: 10 minutes
COOKING TIME: 30 minutes, depending on thickness

1 medium cauliflower
1 teaspoon coriander seeds
1 teaspoon fennel seeds
1 teaspoon turmeric powder
1 teaspoon sweet paprika powder
    (not the super-hot variety)
sprinkle of chilli flakes (optional)
1 garlic clove
4 sprays 1-calorie sunflower oil
    cooking spray

Preheat the oven to 200°C/180°C fan/gas mark 6. Line a baking tray with baking paper.

Trim the cauliflower stalk: leave some young, inner leaves attached. Slice the cauliflower into four 3cm-thick slices. Place the cauliflower steaks on the tray. (Keep the remaining end pieces for another meal.)

Bash all the spices together in a pestle and mortar or grinder, along with the garlic. Rub the cauliflower slices with the spice paste and then spray with the oil. Roast the cauliflower in the oven for about 30 minutes until just tender when tested with the point of a knife.

Cook's Tips

This recipe can be tweaked to use fewer seasonings or any combination of spices you happen to have in the cupboard; for example, curry powder, garam masala, or Moroccan seasoning like ras el hanout.

It also works well with broccoli: cut the head into large florets, season and roast. Alternatively, chill the spiced vegetables and mix with slices of red pepper and cherry tomatoes for a salad.

A spoonful of the Chimichurri Herb Dressing on page 73 will add a slightly sharp herb dressing for the cauliflower, if you just want to serve it on its own as a light lunch.

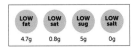

ENERGY 123kcals **PROTEIN** 6.2g | **FAT** 4.7g | **SATURATED FAT** 0.8g
CARBOHYDRATE 15g | **TOTAL SUGARS** 5g | **SALT** 0g | **SODIUM** 4mg | **FIBRE** 9g

Braised Aubergines with Spiced Butterbeans & Crispy Garlic

This easy recipe cuts out 90 per cent of the oil that you would normally use to cook the aubergine. Instead I use water to start the cooking process, then add beans, chilli, garlic and Tabasco to flavour the whole dish, as aubergines can be pretty bland when you remove most of the oil.

Serves 4

PREPARATION TIME: 10 minutes
COOKING TIME: 45 minutes

4 teaspoons olive oil
4 onions, chopped
½ teaspoon chilli flakes
2 large aubergines, cut into
    2cm pieces
400g can butterbeans, drained
    really well
1 teaspoon Tabasco sauce
4 garlic cloves, finely sliced
4 ripe tomatoes, roughly chopped
freshly ground black pepper

Preheat the oven to 200°C/180°C fan/gas mark 6.

Heat 3 teaspoons of the olive oil in a shallow, ovenproof saucepan. Add the onions, chilli flakes and aubergines, mix well and season with a little pepper. Add the butterbeans, 100ml of water and the Tabasco, then cover and bake in the oven for 40 minutes, or until soft and slightly coloured.

Once cooked, remove from the oven and stir well. Heat the remaining teaspoon of oil in a non-stick frying pan, add the garlic and cook over a high heat to get some real colour, until almost burnt. Add the tomatoes and garlic to the aubergines and mix well off the heat. Serve.

Cook's Tip
If you want, you can add some extra protein such as a few prawns or chicken, if you're eating meat, or some sliced boiled egg.

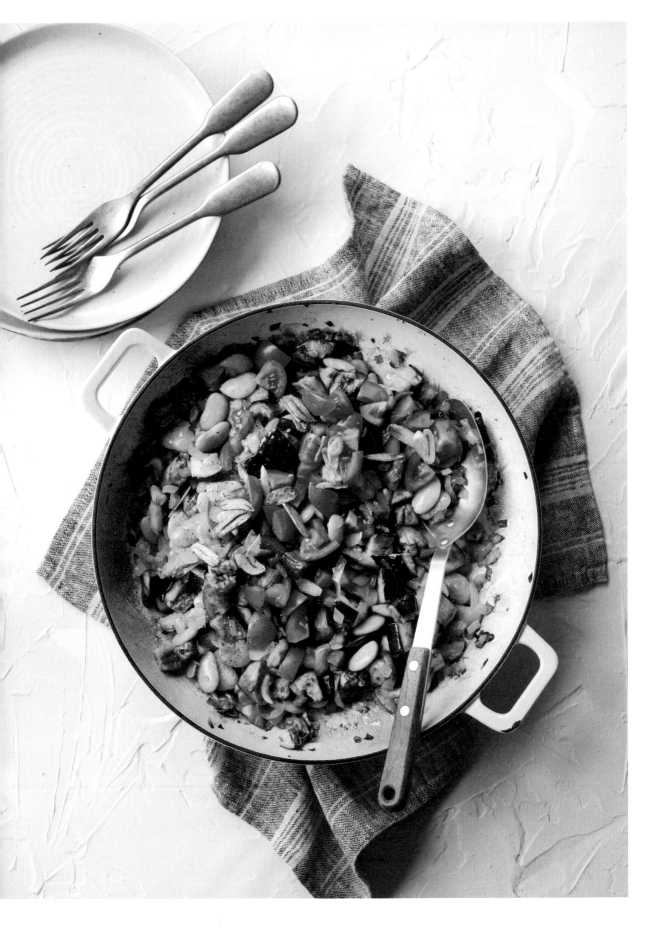

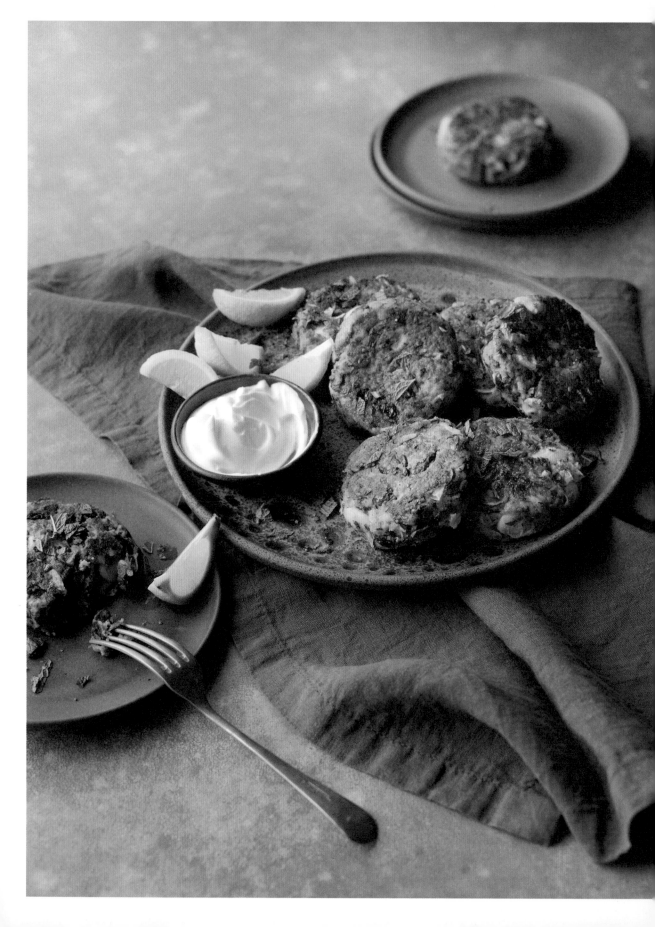

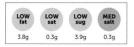

ENERGY 238kcals **PROTEIN** 16g | **FAT** 3.8g | **SATURATED FAT** 0.3g
CARBOHYDRATE 37g | **TOTAL SUGARS** 3.9g | **SALT** 0.3g | **SODIUM** 151mg | **FIBRE** 13g

Moroccan Bean Patties

Really tasty bean patties using spices and fresh herbs to add deep flavour. Again, I add no extra salt here, as there's just a little in the stock. In its place, I add lemon zest and juice.

Serves 4

PREPARATION TIME: 30 minutes
COOKING TIME: 15 minutes

400g can butterbeans, drained well
400g can kidney beans, drained well
2 teaspoons rapeseed oil
2 garlic cloves
1 small onion, finely chopped
1 teaspoon ground cinnamon
1 heaped teaspoon ground cumin
pinch of chilli powder
pinch reduced-salt vegetable
    stock cube dissolved in 125ml
    boiling water
zest and juice of 1 small lemon
2 tablespoons chopped parsley
2 tablespoons chopped mint
3 tablespoons chopped coriander
4 level tablespoons breadcrumbs
1 egg white
freshly ground black pepper

TO SERVE
100g 0%-fat unsweetened yogurt
4 wedges of lemon
2 tablespoons chopped fresh
    mint leaves

Mash the beans lightly with a fork or potato masher; no need to go mad.

Heat 1 teaspoon of the oil in a pan over a low heat and add the garlic and onion. Cook for a few minutes to soften. Add the spices, pepper, stock and lemon zest and juice and cook for 15 minutes, or until almost all the liquid has evaporated. Add the mashed beans and herbs, then remove from the stove and leave to cool.

Once cooled, add enough breadcrumbs and egg white to bring the mix together, then check the seasoning and adjust if needed. Mould into eight patties and flatten slightly, then chill until needed.

Heat a non-stick frying pan over a medium heat and add 1 teaspoon or a spray of oil. Cook the patties for 3–4 minutes on each side. Serve with a little yogurt, a lemon wedge and a sprinkling of fresh chopped mint.

Cook's Tip
Try serving these with a nice small green salad or some veggies on the side.

Nutrition Tip
Butter beans (known as lima beans elsewhere) were a mainstay of the Native American diet. They are an excellent source of protein, fibre, iron and B vitamins.

| LOW fat 3.8g | LOW sat 0.5g | MED sug 13g | MED salt 1g | **ENERGY** 392kcals **PROTEIN** 25g | **FAT** 3.8g | **SATURATED FAT** 0.5g **CARBOHYDRATE** 68g | **TOTAL SUGARS** 13g | **SALT** 1g | **SODIUM** 394mg | **FIBRE** 11g |

Jewelled Five-pulse Dal

Ve

GF

If using gluten-free stock cube and asafoetida

The only thing really to remember here is to soak the pulses overnight first. You can cook them in their dried state, but it can take a long time. The secret is to cook the pulses down until you end up with a thick stew, so the flavour and texture are at their very best; I really dislike dal that is too liquid. I add sultanas, as I once had a dal with them in India; it really adds a nice sweet edge to the final dish. If you can't find asafoetida, try fresh or dried curry leaves; if you don't have either, no problem, it just adds a lovely rounded flavour to the finished dish.

Serves 4

PREPARATION TIME: 30 minutes
COOKING TIME: 40 minutes

100g yellow split peas
100g red lentils
75g green lentils
75g mung beans
75g chickpeas
1 teaspoon bicarbonate of soda
10g reduced-salt vegetable
   stock cube
2 tablespoons tomato purée
½ teaspoon asafoetida
5–6 curry leaves (optional)
50g juicy sultanas
4 tablespoons roughly chopped
   coriander, plus extra to serve

FOR THE ONION SPICE MIX
1 teaspoon rapeseed oil
1 teaspoon cumin seeds
1 teaspoon ground turmeric
6 green cardamom pods, crushed
1 teaspoon garam masala
1 teaspoon fenugreek
½ small green chilli, finely chopped
1 onion, finely chopped
4 garlic cloves
2 tablespoons chopped fresh
   ginger

Wash all the pulses really well in cold water, then pop into a bowl, cover with cold water, add the bicarb and stir well. Cover and place in the fridge overnight.

The next day, rinse really well and place into a clean saucepan. Just cover with cold water and bring to the boil. Skim well, turn the heat down and add the stock cube and tomato purée, asafoetida and curry leaves, if using, and gently simmer for 40–50 minutes. You may need to top up a little with boiling water.

Meanwhile, heat the oil in a non-stick sauté pan. Add the spices and chilli and cook for 1 minute over a high heat. Next add the onion, garlic and ginger, and cook for 5–6 minutes.

Once the pulses are cooked, stir well and break up so the mixture thickens slightly. Add the sultanas and coriander to the pulses and remove from the heat, then stir through the yogurt and leave to infuse for 15 minutes.

Serve in deep bowls topped with the onion spice mix and a little more coriander.

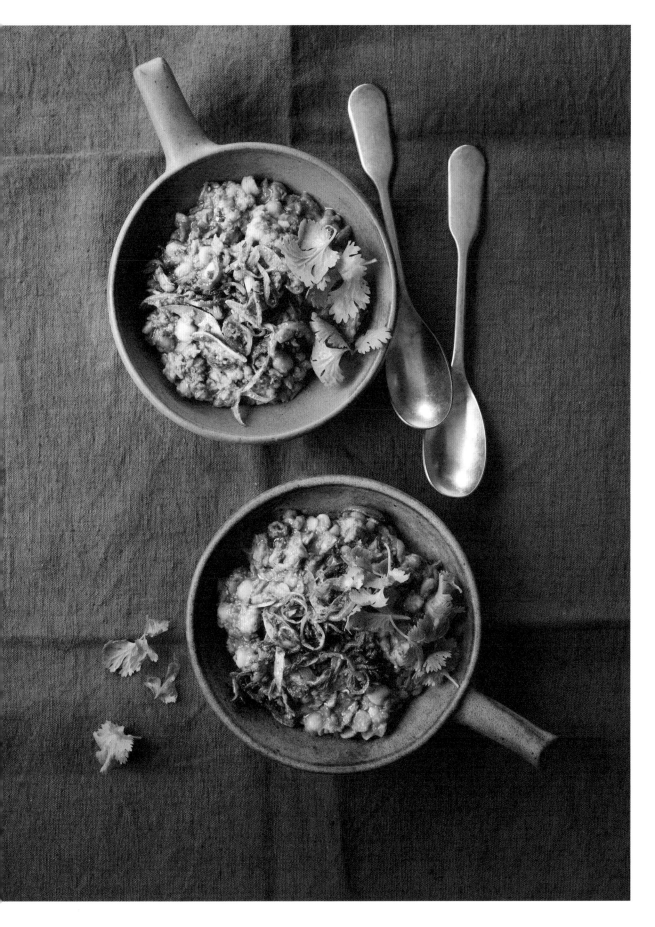

LOW fat 3.8g	LOW sat 0.4g	LOW sug 8.9g	MED salt 0.3g

ENERGY 239kcals **PROTEIN** 13g | **FAT** 3.8g | **SATURATED FAT** 0.4g
CARBOHYDRATE 41g | **TOTAL SUGARS** 8.9g | **SALT** 0.3g | **SODIUM** 114mg | **FIBRE** 8.4g

Five Vegetable Curry

This is a simple, everyday Indian curry with a combination of vegetables you can vary with the seasons. Spinach, Swiss chard or spring greens all work well here.

GF

If using gluten-free curry paste and stock

Serves 4

PREPARATION TIME: 15 minutes
COOKING TIME: 45 minutes

1 teaspoon rapeseed oil
1 onion, chopped
1 red or green pepper, deseeded and sliced
1 squash or sweet potato (150g), peeled and cut into 2cm chunks
200g cauliflower florets
2 teaspoons finely grated fresh ginger
2 garlic cloves, crushed
1 tablespoon mild curry paste (such as balti)
2 teaspoons garam masala (see tip)
227g can chopped tomatoes
1 tablespoon tomato purée
400g can green or brown lentils, rinsed and drained (265g drained weight)
200ml reduced-salt vegetable stock
100g spinach leaves or chard, washed and chopped

TO SERVE
3 tablespoons chopped coriander leaves
4 tablespoons 0%-fat unsweetened yogurt
8 heaped tablespoons (60g) cooked brown basmati rice

Heat the oil in a large pan. Add the onion, pepper and squash or sweet potato and fry for 10 minutes until lightly softened. Add the cauliflower, ginger, garlic and spices and continue to fry for 1 minute.

Add the tomatoes, tomato purée and lentils to the pan and pour over the stock. Bring to the boil, reduce the heat, cover and simmer for 30 minutes or until the vegetables are tender. Stir regularly and add a bit more water if it looks dry.

In the last 10 minutes, stir through the chopped greens and re-cover the pan to wilt them.

Serve with the coriander leaves, two tablespoons each of rice and a spoonful of yogurt.

Cook's Tip

Optional extra spices: it can be difficult to find some spices, so these extras are nice to have but not essential, to add more complex flavours to the curry:

• A few curry leaves simmered with the stock.

• A sprinkle of whole seeds such as 'panch phoran' (also called panch puran), which is an Indian 5 spice blend using whole seeds such as mustard, cumin, fenugreek, fennel and nigella (kalonji).

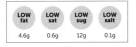

ENERGY 239kcals **PROTEIN** 15g | **FAT** 4.6g | **SATURATED FAT** 0.6g
CARBOHYDRATE 31g | **TOTAL SUGARS** 12g | **SALT** 0.1g | **SODIUM** 28mg | **FIBRE** 22g

Mixed Bean Chilli

If using gluten-free stock cube

There are so many versions of this; you just have to make a favourite and tweak away to suit yourself. There could be such a long list of ingredients for a veggie chilli, adding more depth of flavours, but to make it simpler you can just use more of what you have and less variety. I always find that a good, wide pan, made of something like heavy cast iron, big enough to hold all the ingredients, cooks a better result in the end.

Serves 4

PREPARATION TIME: 15 minutes
COOKING TIME: 45–60 minutes

2 teaspoons rapeseed oil
1 red onion, finely chopped
1 garlic clove, crushed
1 courgette, cut into chunky dice
1 red or green pepper, deseeded and chopped
1 medium carrot, peeled and chopped
2 teaspoons dried spice mix (or 1 teaspoon each: ground cumin; spiced smoked paprika or chilli powder to taste; and crushed cumin and coriander seeds, optional)
400g can chopped tomatoes
15g sliced dried mushrooms, soaked in 75ml boiling water (optional)
400g can kidney beans, drained and rinsed
400g can black beans, drained and rinsed
400ml reduced-salt vegetable stock
1 teaspoon balsamic vinegar (optional)

Heat a large heavy pan with the oil and sauté the onion until soft, about 8–10 minutes. Add the garlic and the vegetables and cook, stirring, for about a further 5 minutes. Keep the heat fairly high so the vegetables don't steam.

Stir in the spice mix, tomatoes, mushrooms, if using, and both beans. Top up with vegetable stock and vinegar, if using, and simmer gently for about 45 minutes, half covered with the lid. Keep an eye on the pan to check if the liquid is getting too low, and give it a stir every now and again.

Cook's Tip

Serve with freshly ground black pepper and 3 tablespoons of rice per person; choose wholegrain, basmati, brown, red or black rice.

Or serve with jacket sweet potatoes: wash the sweet potatoes well and bake in the oven for 1 hour or until soft and with crunchy skins. If you are choosing this option, then transfer the chilli from the hob to the oven, to cook at the same time instead of simmering for 45 minutes.

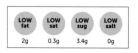

ENERGY 100kcals **PROTEIN** 6.6g | **FAT** 2g | **SATURATED FAT** 0.3g
CARBOHYDRATE 10g | **TOTAL SUGARS** 3.4g | **SALT** 0g | **SODIUM** 3mg | **FIBRE** 12g

Mexican Refried Black Beans

This could make a sharing plate dip, or you can crack in an egg for a tasty lunch. The Spanish name for refried beans is 'frijoles refritos', which actually means 'well-fried', not 'fried again'. Refried beans are a staple in Mexican cuisine, consisting of cooked beans that are mashed and seasoned. Original Mexican recipes use pinto beans cooked with lots of lard and salt. In some parts of Mexico, black beans are more common to use than pinto, but you can use red kidney beans or a mix of beans instead. I've replaced the lard with tomatoes to make it a bit healthier.

Serves 4

PREPARATION TIME: 15 minutes
COOKING TIME: 20 minutes

1 teaspoon olive oil
1 small red onion, finely chopped
1 garlic clove, crushed
225g can chopped tomatoes in juice
400g can black beans, drained and
    rinsed (240g drained weight)
½ teaspoon ground cumin
pinch of chilli powder, to taste
½ teaspoon dried oregano

Heat the oil in a medium saucepan over a medium heat. Add the onion and cook for 8–10 minutes until softened.

Add the garlic, stirring for another minute, and then mix in the tomatoes, beans, spices and oregano. Simmer until the tomatoes begin to reduce and the liquid thickens slightly. Break up the beans and mash them lightly, then simmer for a further 5 minutes, stirring constantly. Remove from the heat.

Refried beans can be served hot, at room temperature or cold, and as a main dish, side dish, filling, garnish or dip.

Cook's Tip
Instead of serving with traditional nachos and tacos, which are high in salt and calories from oil, try my recipe for Savoury Socca Pancakes on page 89. Fill the flatbread and roll it up like a burrito or tear the hot flatbread to eat with the refried beans as a dip with some salsa. Just mix together the following ingredients and serve:

2 large tomatoes, chopped
a small handful of fresh coriander or basil leaves, chopped
1 spring onion, sliced
1 mild jalapeño chilli, sliced very thin
1 lime, quartered

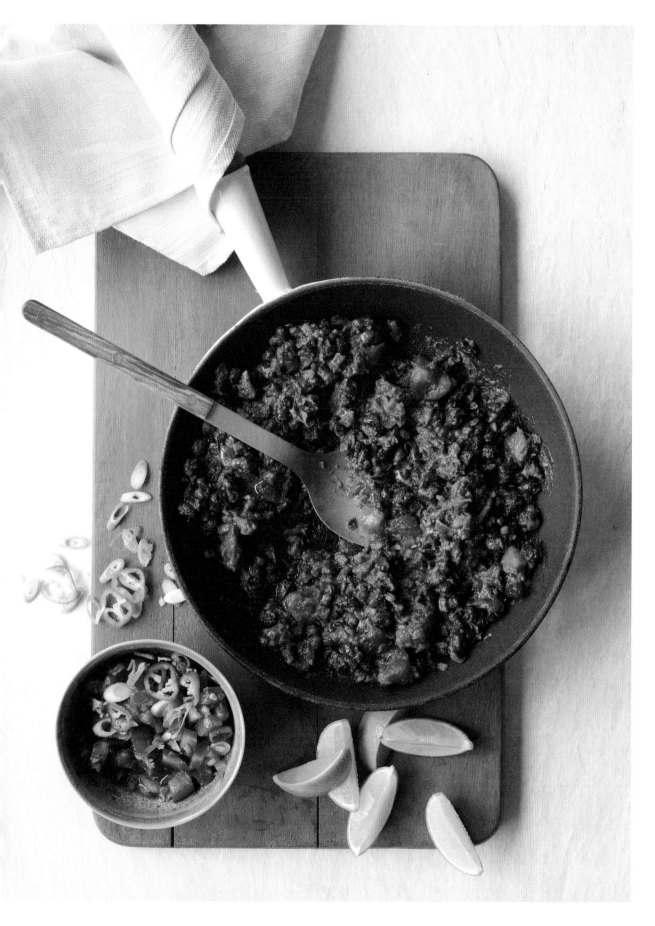

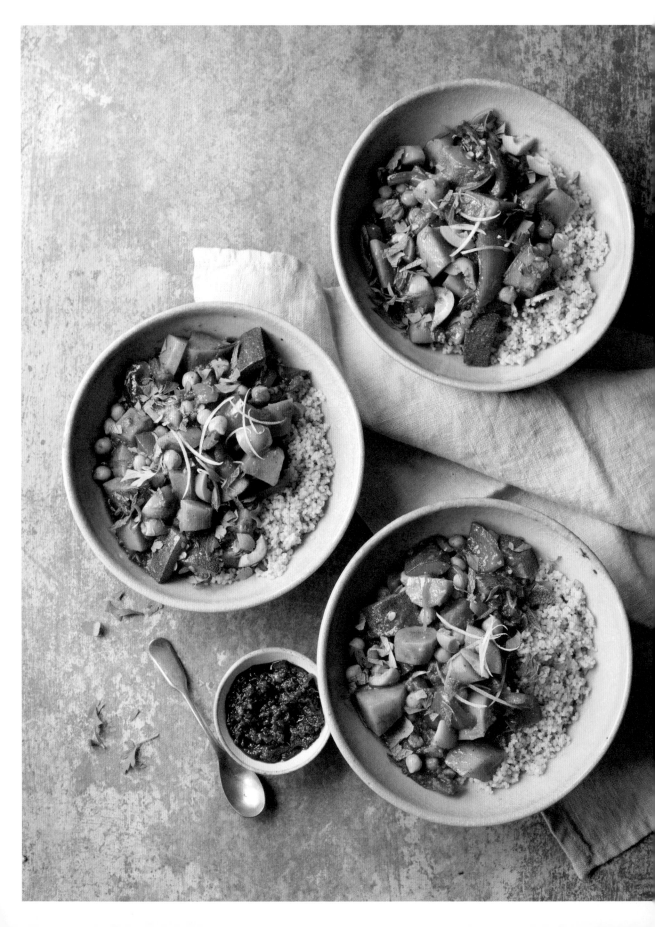

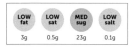

ENERGY 231kcals **PROTEIN** 8.5g | **FAT** 3g | **SATURATED FAT** 0.5g

CARBOHYDRATE 45g | **TOTAL SUGARS** 23g | **SALT** 0.1g | **SODIUM** 48mg | **FIBRE** 12g

Vegetable Tagine with Chickpeas

If using gluten-free stock cube

Tagine is named after the distinctive cone-shaped dish in which it is made. Traditionally made from glazed clay and used for cooking over coals, tagines came from the Berber culture, and are now used throughout North Africa but most commonly in Morocco. A sweet and sour combination of cumin, coriander and cinnamon, as well as other spices and sometimes chilli, is the hallmark of a classic tagine.

Serves 4

PREPARATION TIME: 15 minutes
COOKING TIME: 1 hour

1 teaspoon rapeseed oil
800g prepared vegetables such as:
　1 red onion, sliced
　1 courgette, cut into small chunks
　1 medium carrot, peeled and cut
　　into chunks
　1 red pepper, deseeded and cubed
　1 small sweet potato, peeled and
　　cut into small chunks
1 garlic clove, crushed
1 teaspoon grated fresh ginger
1 tablespoon ras el hanout spice
　mix
¼ teaspoon cumin or coriander
　seeds
1 tablespoon lemon juice
400g can chickpeas, drained
　and rinsed
50g dates, pitted and quartered
　(or use dried apricots)
200ml reduced-salt vegetable stock
400g tomatoes, roughly chopped

TO SERVE (OPTIONAL)
1 teaspoon finely sliced lemon rind
4 green olives, pitted and halved
2 tablespoons herbs, roughly
　chopped (such as parsley,
　coriander leaves and mint leaves)
200g steamed couscous
2 teaspoons harissa paste

Preheat the oven to 180°C/160°C fan/gas mark 4.

Heat the oil in a large, heavy-based pan over a medium heat. Add the onions and cook for 5 minutes until soft and starting to colour, stirring occasionally.

Add the courgette, carrot, pepper and sweet potato and continue to cook for another 5 minutes.

Next add the garlic, fresh ginger and spices and cook for a couple of minutes until fragrant.

Add the rest of the ingredients and bring to a simmer. Cover with a lid and transfer to the oven. Bake for 45 minutes to 1 hour until reduced down and soft. Alternatively, you can do this on the hob; lower the heat and check it isn't catching on the bottom.

To serve, stir in lemon rind and garnish each plate with olives and chopped herbs, and serve with steamed couscous and a dollop of harissa for spice.

Nutrition Tip
Chickpeas have been grown in Middle Eastern countries for thousands of years. Also known as garbanzo beans, they are high in protein and a rich source of B vitamins, zinc and fibre.

LOW fat	LOW sat	LOW sug	MED salt
4.7g	0.9g	4.7g	0.3g

ENERGY 225kcals **PROTEIN** 5.2g | **FAT** 4.7g | **SATURATED FAT** 0.9g
CARBOHYDRATE 47g | **TOTAL SUGARS** 4.7g | **SALT** 0.3g | **SODIUM** 124mg | **FIBRE** 7.1g

Celeriac Risotto

GF
If using gluten-free stock cube

I love this recipe as it shows you can produce a great, hearty main course with no meat or fish protein at all. The only real pain I suppose is the cutting of the celeriac; I blanch the cubes purely as I think you get a better end texture. I have also made this with swede, turnip and parsnips instead of the celeriac. No salt is added as I use a stock cube. I sometimes add a little extra veg like baby spinach or even a can of beans to bulk it out.

Serves 4

PREPARATION TIME: 30 minutes
COOKING TIME: 15–20 minutes

1 medium celeriac (450g), trimmed and cut into roughly 5mm cubes
1 litre boiling water
2 garlic cloves, finely chopped
10g reduced-salt vegetable stock cube
½ teaspoon ground turmeric
1 onion, finely chopped
200g Arborio rice
4 tablespoons roughly chopped chives
1–2 tablespoons low-fat crème fraîche or unsweetened yogurt (optional)
freshly ground black pepper

Place the chopped celeriac into a saucepan and add the water, garlic, stock cube and turmeric.

Bring to the boil, then simmer for 30 seconds. Strain into a bowl reserving all the stock.

Place the blanched celeriac and bits and bobs into a large sauté pan, ensuring to get all the garlic. Add the onion and rice and mix well.

Bring to the boil, then start adding the hot stock. Turn down the heat, stirring occasionally, as you keep adding the hot stock; you will see the rice swell and the celeriac start to soften and cook. The rice may start to stick as the starch is released, so turn the heat down.

Once all the stock is added and the rice and celeriac are only just cooked, remove from the heat, add a little ground pepper, cover and leave for 5 minutes.

After 5 minutes, remove the lid, add the chives and crème fraîche or yogurt, stir well and then serve.

Nutrition Tip
Closely related to celery, parsley and parsnips, celeriac is a nutritional powerhouse packed with fibre and vitamins B6, C and K. It's also a good source of minerals such as phosphorus, potassium and manganese.

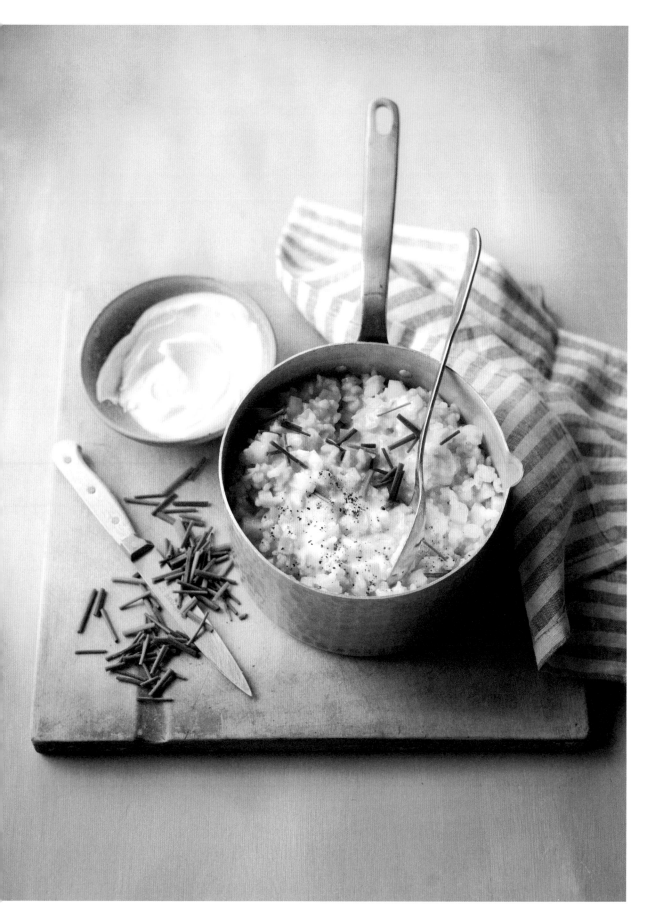

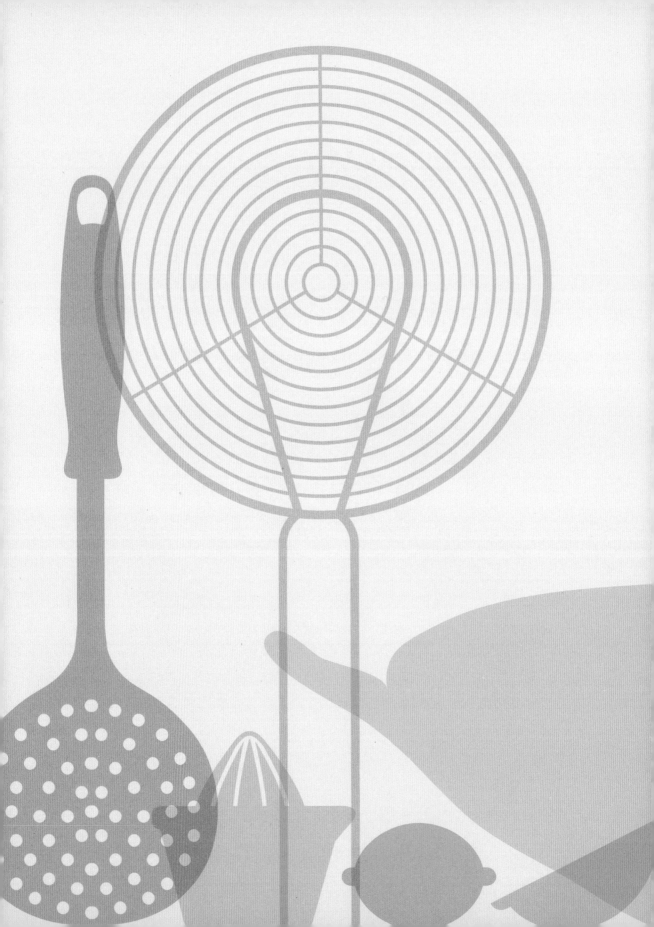

Fish
& Seafood

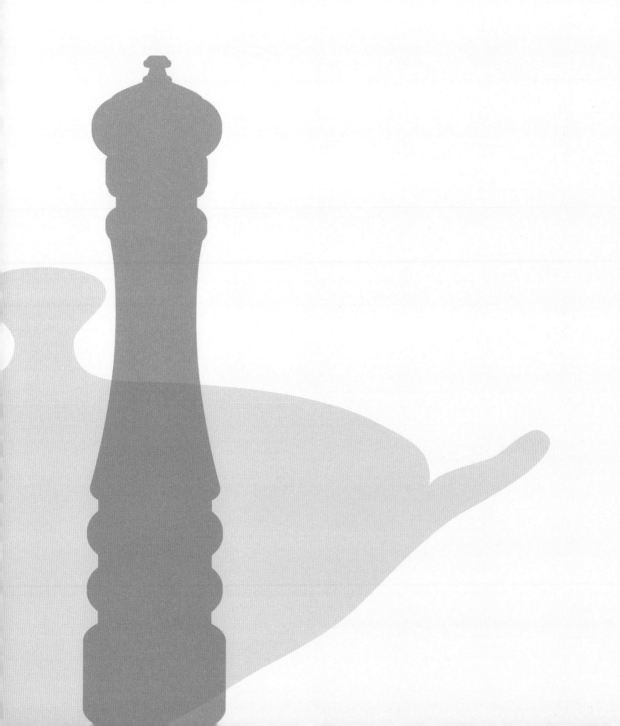

ENERGY 230kcals PROTEIN 17g | FAT 14g | SATURATED FAT 2.5g
CARBOHYDRATE 10g | TOTAL SUGARS 2g | SALT 0.29g | SODIUM 135mg | FIBRE 2g

MED fat 14g | MED sat 2.5g | LOW sug 2g | LOW salt 0.29g

Tandoori Salmon

This is a great alternative to serve with the Fish Tacos (opposite). Fish contains much less saturated fat than meat, and salmon in particular is full of omega-3 fatty acids and vitamin D.

Serves 4

PREPARATION TIME: 5 minutes
COOKING TIME: 8 minutes

300g skinless, boneless salmon fillet
2 tablespoons low-fat unsweetened
  yogurt
2 teaspoons tandoori paste
4 lemon wedges

Cut the salmon into large cubes and remove any bones.

Mix the yogurt and tandoori paste together in a bowl, then add the salmon and coat gently.

Grill the salmon pieces for 5–8 minutes or until cooked through, turning halfway through. Serve with the lemon wedges.

Nutrition Tip
As well as being rich in omega-3 fatty acids, salmon is a good source of protein, B vitamins, potassium and selenium.

MED fat	MED sat	LOW sug	MED salt
4.7g	0.8g	0.7g	0.1g

Fish Tacos

These tacos can be an easy lunch or a crowd pleaser when scaled up. The fish can easily be adapted for many filling options (see the recipe for Tandoori Salmon opposite) and you can take advantage of seasonal produce for the salad.

Serves 4

PREPARATION TIME: 10 minutes
COOKING TIME: 5 minutes

4 firm white fish fillets, skinned (approx. 100g each; frozen and defrosted is fine)
2 teaspoons homemade jerk seasoning (see tip)
1 garlic clove, crushed
8 sprays 1-calorie vegetable oil cooking spray

TO SERVE
4 wholegrain corn tortillas or taco shells
small bag mixed salad
30g red cabbage, very finely sliced (optional)
1 lime, cut into 4 wedges
4 teaspoons low-fat unsweetened live yogurt
fresh chilli, chopped, or a few drops chilli sauce

If you are using frozen, defrosted fish, drain any excess water and pat dry. Mix together the spices with the garlic and rub this mixture over the fish fillets to coat.

Spray a heavy-based, non-stick frying pan with the oil and heat over a medium–high heat. Cook the fish on each side, until the fillets colour and flake when pulled with a fork: this might be only a couple of minutes if the fillets are thin. Put the cooked, flaked fish in a bowl and keep warm.

Warm the tortillas or taco shells, add a handful of salad leaves, then divide the fish between them. Top with the red cabbage, if using, a squeeze of lime juice, a teaspoon of yogurt and some chilli.

Cook's Tip
Make your own jerk seasoning mix with ½ teaspoon each smoked, hot paprika, ground cumin and ground allspice, and a tiny pinch of thyme.

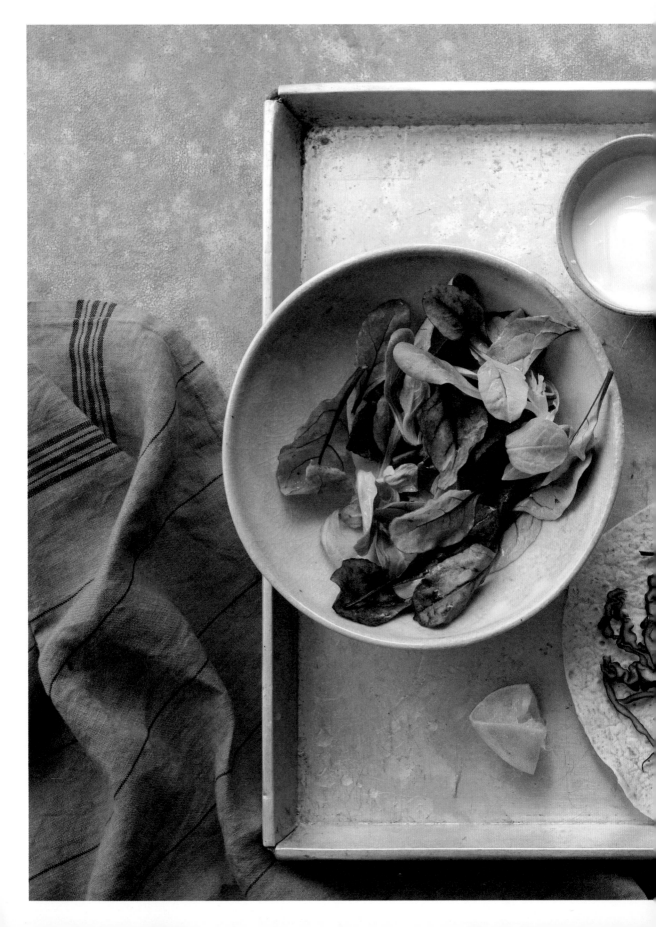

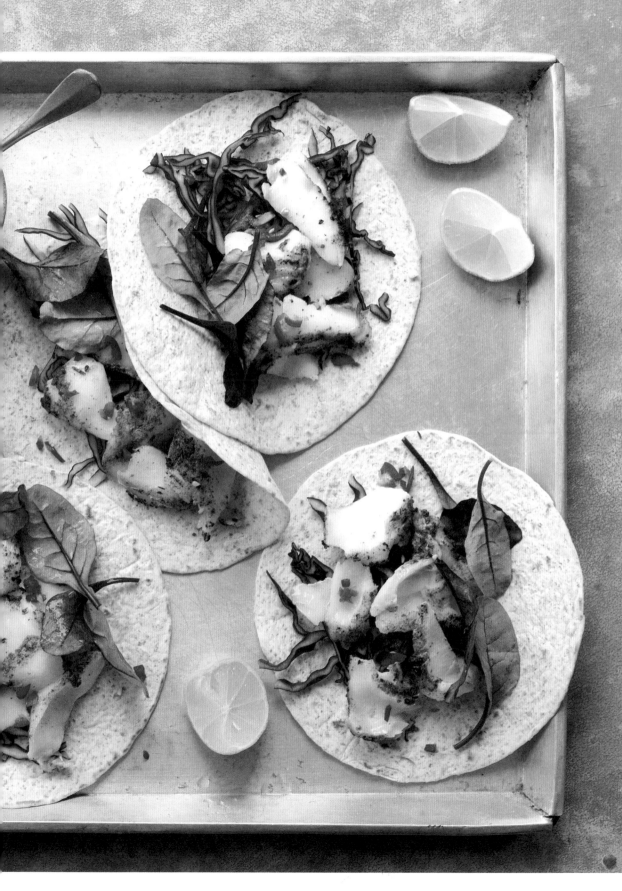

ENERGY 298kcals **PROTEIN** 20g | **FAT** 20g | **SATURATED FAT** 4g

CARBOHYDRATE 8.6g | **TOTAL SUGARS** 7.7g | **SALT** 0.4g | **SODIUM** 171mg | **FIBRE** 3.8g

Sweet Pickled Mackerel

GF

If using gluten-free stock cube

This method of cooking fish is very trendy at the moment, but in fact, it has been around for centuries. Basically it's a lightly pickled fish dish with vegetables. It's best left for a couple of days in the fridge after it's cooked, to get the best flavour out of the fish. I'm using mackerel here as it's a great summer fish and good value for money.

Serves 4

PREPARATION TIME: 15 minutes
COOKING TIME: 15 minutes

1 teaspoon olive oil
4 large mackerel fillets (400g), transparent skin removed and boned
2 small onions, very finely chopped
2 large carrots, peeled and cut into very small cubes
1 courgette, cut into very small cubes
200ml white wine vinegar
½ × 10g reduced-salt fish stock cube
2 garlic cloves, crushed
½ small red chilli, very finely chopped
½ teaspoon granulated sweetener
juice of 1 lemon
freshly ground black pepper

Heat a large, non-stick frying pan, add the oil and swirl around.

Season the mackerel fillets with a little ground pepper, and then add to the pan, skin-side down. Cook for 3 minutes until the skin starts to blister. Remove the fish from the pan and place in an earthenware or glass dish.

Add the onions, carrots and courgette to the pan, then add the vinegar, 300ml of cold water and the stock cube, garlic, chilli and sweetener. Bring to the boil and then turn down the heat and simmer for 5 minutes. Check the seasoning and adjust if necessary.

Pour this hot pickle mixture over the fish, then pour over the lemon juice and cover the dish with clingfilm. Leave to cool and chill in the fridge for up to 2 days.

Serve chilled or at room temperature, with green salad and little crusty wholemeal sourdough.

Nutrition Tip

An oily fish rich in the polyunsaturated fats known as omega-3s, mackerel is a good source of protein and B vitamins, particularly vitamin B12, as well as the mineral selenium, which can help protect our cells against damaging free-radicals.

LOW fat	LOW sat	LOW sug	MED salt	**ENERGY** 285kcals **PROTEIN** 22g	**FAT** 7g	**SATURATED FAT** 2.4g
7g	2.4g	10g	0.7g	**CARBOHYDRATE** 35g	**TOTAL SUGARS** 10g	**SALT** 0.7g	**SODIUM** 295mg	**FIBRE** 3.7g

Potato, Herb, Tuna & Rice Frittata (GF)

I have always enjoyed canned tuna; it is very versatile and very good for you. My grandma loved the stuff, and would eat it with pickled or raw onions. Like all canned fish, it needs little to no cooking; all you do is warm it gently so it doesn't dry out. I first cooked a version of this on 'This Morning' and it went down well. I like to eat this sort of food in front of the television, or if I'm on my own and can't be bothered to cook a full-blown meal; it is so simple to make.

Serves 4

PREPARATION TIME: 30 minutes
COOKING TIME: 15 minutes

1 teaspoon olive oil
225g cooked sweet potatoes, cut into slices (bake, wrapped in foil, in a moderate oven for 30 minutes)
1 small onion, very finely chopped
185g can tuna in water, drained
250g sachet microwavable wholegrain or brown basmati rice, heated
2 eggs
4 egg whites
1 teaspoon dried oregano
2 tablespoons fresh parsley, chopped
25g mature Cheddar, very finely grated (optional)
freshly ground black pepper

Set the grill to high or heat the oven to 200°C/180°C fan/gas mark 6.

Heat the oil in a non-stick, ovenproof frying pan, and add the potato slices, overlapping slightly. Cook for a few seconds until they take on a little colour. Sprinkle over the raw onion, tuna and cooked rice.

In a bowl, whisk together the eggs and whites, oregano and parsley, then add a little black pepper. Pour this over the potato mixture, then sprinkle over the cheese, if using. Place the pan under the grill or in the oven until risen and set, about 6–8 minutes.

Invert onto a plate and cut into wedges; serve hot or cold.

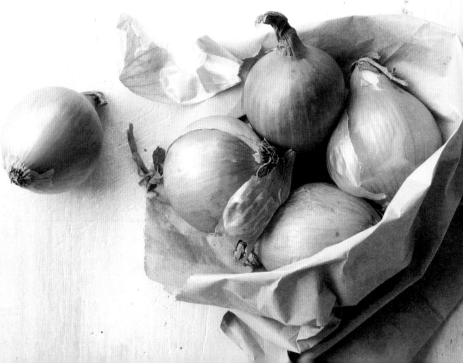

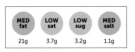

ENERGY 453kcals **PROTEIN** 33g | **FAT** 21g | **SATURATED FAT** 3.7g
CARBOHYDRATE 36g | **TOTAL SUGARS** 3.2g | **SALT** 1.1g | **SODIUM** 432mg | **FIBRE** 5g

Salmon in Miso Broth with Black Rice and Braised Greens

GF

If using gluten-free miso paste

Miso is made from soy beans and often rice or other grains, left to ferment. Black rice is worth seeking out, for its texture, flavour and nutritional value: it has the same kind of anthocyanin pigments as blueberries, is high in heart-healthy polyphenols and has more fibre and protein than white or brown rice. It does take ages to cook and can be expensive, so cook ahead and keep some in the freezer. Or use brown or red rice to add healthy fibre, vitamins and minerals to your meal.

Serves 2

PREPARATION TIME: 10 minutes
COOKING TIME: 50 minutes

75g black rice
80g sprouting broccoli (thicker
  stalks thinly sliced lengthways)
80g sugar snap peas or mangetout
80g pak choi, finely shredded
250g salmon fillets, skinned, boned
  and cut into 3mm cubes
1 tablespoon white miso paste
chives or a sprinkling of dried
  seaweed flakes, to serve

To cook the rice, bring 600ml of water to the boil in a small pan, add the black rice, reduce the heat and simmer gently for about 40 minutes until the rice is tender (it has a unique, firm texture, so it won't be soft). Half-cover the pan during cooking and check on it regularly in case it froths up and spills over or needs a top up with water.

Heat 300ml of water in a large pan. Add the sprouting broccoli to the pan first and simmer for 1 minute, then add the sugar snap peas or mangetout and the pak choi. Add the salmon and poach gently in the broth for 3–4 minutes or until just flaking. Keep the heat low, to a simmer; the trick is to keep the cooking brief, the veg crunchy and not overcook the fish. Fast and simple is the best way to cook most fish.

Remove the heat and, lastly, whisk the miso paste into the hot but not boiling water, salmon and veg. The rice should have absorbed most of its water, so to serve, just spoon it between two large soup bowls. Ladle the broth, salmon and greens onto the rice and snip some chives or seaweed over the top.

Nutrition Tip
Miso is high in salt but protein- and nutrient-rich, and varies in colour, from creamy white to dark brown, which signifies the intensity and saltiness of its flavour. White miso is the mildest and least salty, but use it sparingly; adding it last, with the pan off the heat, preserves the beneficial fermentation bacteria (probiotics).

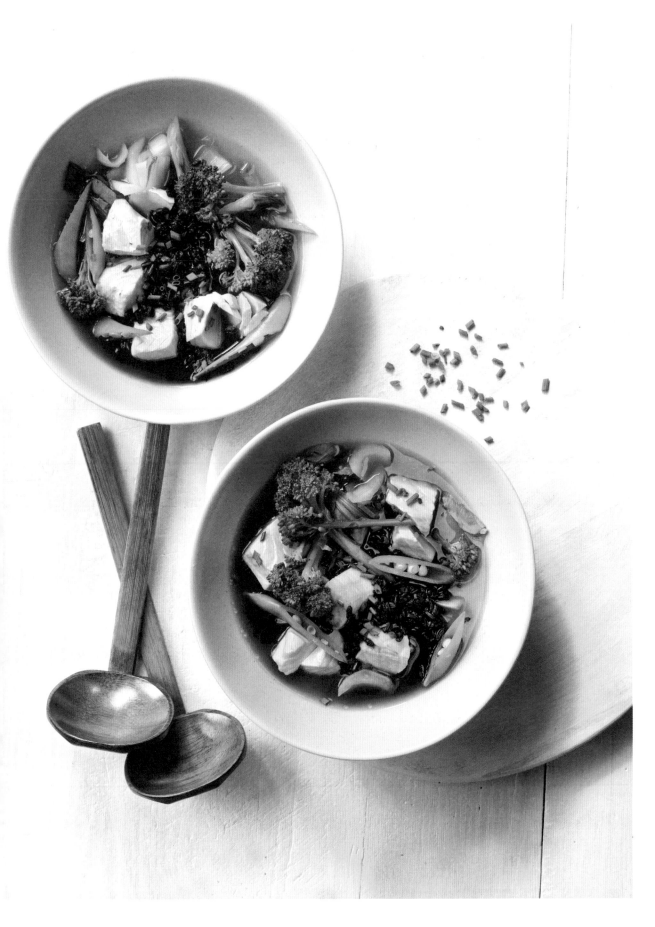

LOW fat 2.3g	LOW sat 0.2g	LOW sug 1g	MED salt 0.4g

ENERGY 125kcals **PROTEIN** 20g | **FAT** 2.3g | **SATURATED FAT** 0.2g
CARBOHYDRATE 6.6g | **TOTAL SUGARS** 1g | **SALT** 0.4g | **SODIUM** 168mg | **FIBRE** 1.5g

Spiced Fish Cakes

GF

If using gluten-free curry paste

Fish cakes can make a tasty alternative burger in a bun but are often deep-fried and coated in crumbs. If you keep the mix quite firm, they can be oven-baked or pan-fried in a good, solid, non-stick pan. I prefer to keep bigger chunks of fish in the mix for extra texture. A few peeled raw prawns, roughly chopped, substituted for the same weight of fish would be nice to fold through the fish paste, but mind the salt level.

Serves 2

PREPARATION TIME: 10 minutes
COOKING TIME: 15 minutes

200g firm raw white fish fillets, skinned and boned
1–2 teaspoons curry paste (Indian or Thai)
2 spring onions, finely chopped
finely grated zest of ½ lemon
¼ large red chilli, finely chopped (optional)
1 tablespoon gram (chickpea) flour

Cut the fish into chunks and place into a food-processor with the curry paste, spring onions and lemon zest and pulse until it is mixed well but not a smooth paste. Scrape the mixture into a small bowl and fold through the chilli, if using, (the curry paste might be spicy enough for you already). Alternatively, chop everything together by hand.

Form two burgers from the fish mixture, no more than 2.5cm thick, and set aside to chill in the fridge for at least 30 minutes, or until ready to cook.

Preheat the oven to 200°C/180°C fan/gas mark 6.

When you're ready, place the burgers onto a tray lined with greaseproof paper or foil. Bake until cooked through, about 15 minutes.

See the Blueprint Burgers on page 140 for serving ideas.

Cook's Tip
You could also make this with salmon, including canned salmon: plenty of omega-3. Look for sustainable fish like pollock, which is perfectly good to use from frozen if drained, squeezed and dried well after defrosting, and it's a bit cheaper.

LOW fat	LOW sat	LOW sug	MED salt
5g	1g	12g	0.4g

Really Easy Seafood & Tomato Stew

GF

If using gluten-free stock cube

I really have no problem using frozen seafood bags as long as they are of good quality. Generally that means buying by price: the more expensive they are, the better they seem to be. If there is a downside, it's that sometimes the seafood can be a little gritty. But the plus side is that it's convenient and always available from the freezer. Here, I make a very simple tomato base to which I add a little sweetener to balance out the acidity of the tomatoes. Real one-pot food.

Serves 2

PREPARATION TIME: 10 minutes
COOKING TIME: 35 minutes

1 teaspoon olive oil
2 small onions, finely chopped
2 garlic cloves, chopped
400g can chopped tomatoes
   in juice
10g reduced-salt fish stock cube
1 teaspoon granulated sweetener
2 tablespoons any vinegar
450g bag mixed frozen seafood
4 tablespoons chopped parsley
freshly ground black pepper

Heat the oil in a deep saucepan, then add the onion and garlic, and cook for 2–3 minutes.

Add the tomatoes, stock cube, sweetener, vinegar and some pepper. Add the frozen fish, then fill the tomato can to the top with water and add this to the pan, then bring the pan to a boil. Simmer for 15–20 minutes or until thick and really tasty.

Finally, add the parsley and check the seasoning; adjust if needed.

Nutrition Tip

Tomatoes get their red skin from the antioxidant lycopene, which is easier for the body to absorbed when tomatoes are cooked. Lycopene is linked to balancing free radical levels in the body, which can help protect against disease.

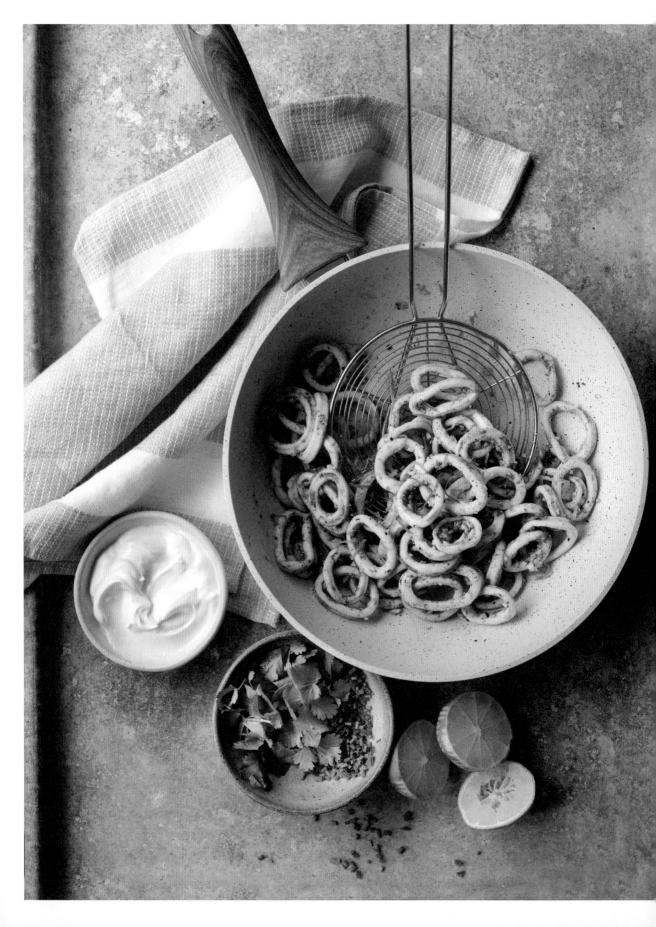

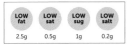

ENERGY 111kcals **PROTEIN** 20g | **FAT** 2.5g | **SATURATED FAT** 0.5g

CARBOHYDRATE 2.4g | **TOTAL SUGARS** 1g | **SALT** 0.2g | **SODIUM** 133mg | **FIBRE** 0g

LOW fat	LOW sat	LOW sug	LOW salt
2.5g	0.5g	1g	0.2g

Sautéed Squid with Yogurt & Lime

The first thing you need to do here is split all the ingredients in half (apart from the yogurt) as you are going to cook in two batches. This makes the job a lot easier and keeps the heat in the wok or large pan. This is essential for getting a nice colour on the squid; this also stops it from boiling. Ensure you pat the squid dry on kitchen towel. I have no problem with using frozen squid; in fact I think the freezing process helps by slightly tenderising the flesh, especially with larger ones. I use no salt in this dish, but instead rely on the spices, ginger, garlic and lime, to boost the flavour.

Serves 4

PREPARATION TIME: 30 minutes
COOKING TIME: 10–15 minutes

½ teaspoon rapeseed oil
450g cleaned squid, cut into
    1cm slices
½ teaspoon freshly ground black
    pepper
½ teaspoon garam masala
2 tablespoons very finely chopped
    fresh ginger
2 garlic cloves, very finely chopped
finely grated zest and juice of
    2 large limes
100g 0%-fat unsweetened yogurt
4 tablespoons chopped chives
4 tablespoons chopped coriander

Heat a large, non-stick wok or frying pan, then add ¼ teaspoon of oil and swirl around. Season all the squid with the pepper and the garam masala.

Add half the squid to the hot wok or pan, and sauté quickly for 1 minute. Add half the ginger and garlic and cook for a further 1 minute, then add half the lime zest and juice. Spoon into a bowl and keep warm. Repeat the process then spoon into the bowl along with the first batch.

Stir through the yogurt, chives and coriander and serve.

Nutrition Tip

Squid is a good source of vitamin B12 as well as potassium, iron, phosphorus and copper.

ENERGY 113kcals **PROTEIN** 11g | **FAT** 2.4g | **SATURATED FAT** 0.4g
CARBOHYDRATE 13g | **TOTAL SUGARS** 9g | **SALT** 0.5g | **SODIUM** 199mg | **FIBRE** 4.7g

Spicy Cauliflower Rice with Prawns & Baby Spinach

GF
If using gluten-free soy sauce

Cauliflower has become very popular recently, from pizza to the old reworked favourite cauli cheese. It can work really well in certain dishes, but to get any real flavour, you need to roast or cook really hard to drive off a lot of the moisture and intensify the flavour. Every dish I cook with cauliflower I roast or sauté first. I also apply the same rule to pumpkin and squash. The smaller the florets when you roast, the drier the rough purée will be, so don't purée to a smooth paste.

Serves 4

PREPARATION TIME: 30 minutes
COOKING TIME: 30–40 minutes

1 cauliflower (approx. 500–600g), cut into small florets (the smaller the better)
1 teaspoon rapeseed oil
½ teaspoon freshly ground black pepper
2 red onions, chopped
2 garlic cloves, finely chopped
2 tablespoons chopped fresh ginger
½ teaspoon finely chopped fresh red chilli
150g bag fresh spinach, washed really well
120g cooked or fresh prawns, finely chopped
2 teaspoons reduced-salt soy sauce

Preheat the oven to 220°C/200°C fan/gas mark 7.

In a pan or tray, coat the cauliflower with the oil and a little ground pepper. Mix well, then pop into the oven and cook for 15 minutes or until you get a nice colour on the cauliflower. You may have to turn occasionally.

Meanwhile, heat a non-stick frying pan over a medium heat and add the onions, garlic, ginger and chilli. Dry-fry (it does work) and stir to take on a little colour for about 4–5 minutes.

Once the cauliflower is well roasted, remove from the oven. Tip into a food-processor and blitz until you have a breadcrumb texture, but don't go mad; you don't want a purée. Add this to the onions and garlic and cook until nice and dry.

Add the spinach, chopped prawns and soy sauce and cook for 2–3 minutes until the spinach has wilted down. Serve in deep bowls.

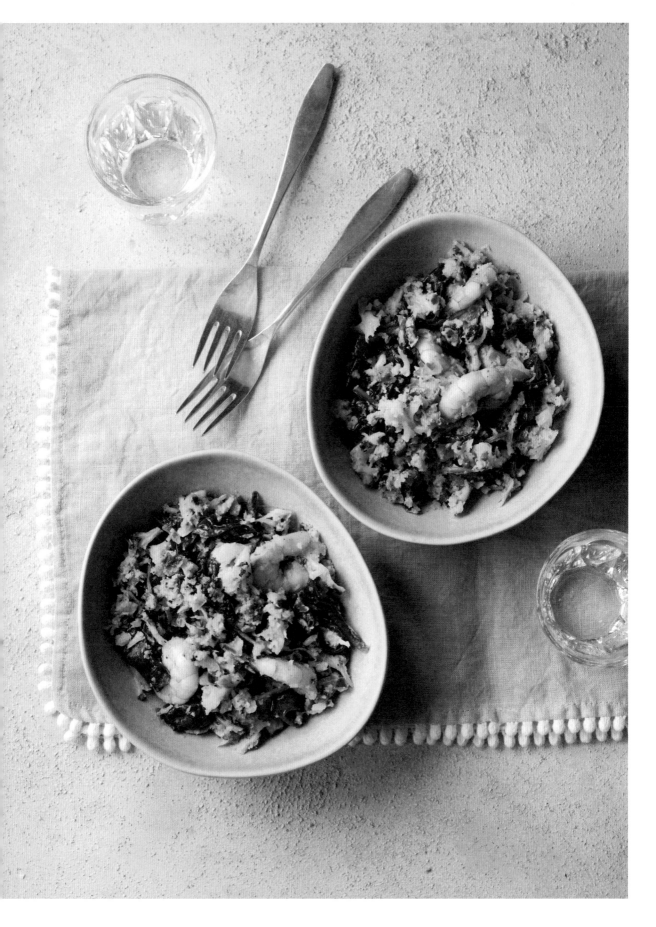

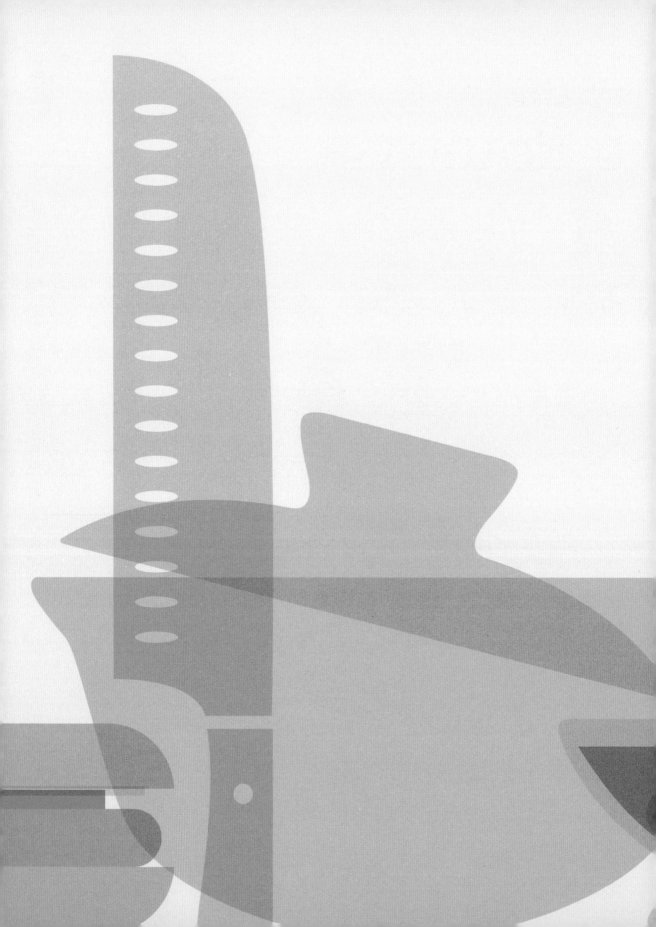

Meat & Poultry

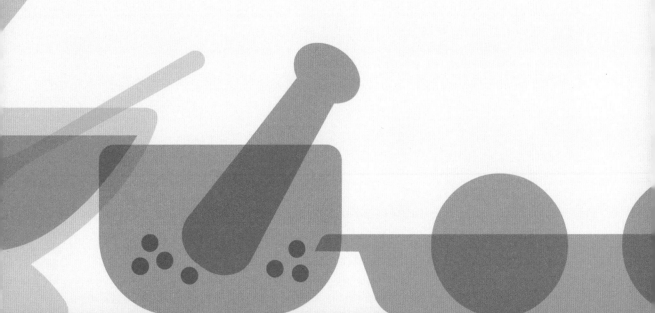

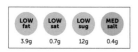

ENERGY 245kcals **PROTEIN** 26g | **FAT** 3.9g | **SATURATED FAT** 0.7g
CARBOHYDRATE 22g | **TOTAL SUGARS** 12g | **SALT** 0.4g | **SODIUM** 148mg | **FIBRE** 11g

Spring Braised Chicken with Little Gem, Peas & Beans

I really like braising lettuce, not only for the texture but also for the colour it brings to the dish. You can use a red lettuce such as radicchio, or even chicory, though they do have a slightly bitter edge. You can, of course, use only one chicken breast or even remove the chicken altogether; just replace it with more vegetables to bulk out the dish and swap in a vegetable stock cube to make it vegetarian.

Serves 4

PREPARATION TIME: 25 minutes
COOKING TIME: 35–40 minutes

1 teaspoon rapeseed oil
2 medium chicken breasts, skinned and cut into thick slices
2 Little Gem lettuce, cut into quarters
2 red onions, finely chopped
4 garlic cloves, finely chopped
1 tablespoon wholemeal flour
pinch of chicken stock cube
200g thin baby carrots, washed really well (you can blanch first, if you want)
200g frozen peas
200g frozen broad beans
freshly ground black pepper

Preheat the oven to 200°C/180°C fan/gas mark 6.

Heat the oil in a large, ovenproof, non-stick sauté pan, then add the chicken and brown well for about 10 minutes. Remove the chicken and then quickly brown the lettuce wedges in the pan, then remove.

Add the onions and garlic and, again, quickly sauté, then add a little flour to soak up the oil.

Add 600ml of water and the stock cube and bring to a simmer, then add the chicken, carrots, peas, beans and lettuce. Bring to a simmer, cover and pop into the oven for 25 minutes, or until the chicken and carrots are just cooked.

Nutrition Tips
Chicken is a rich source of carnosine which can support the immune system.

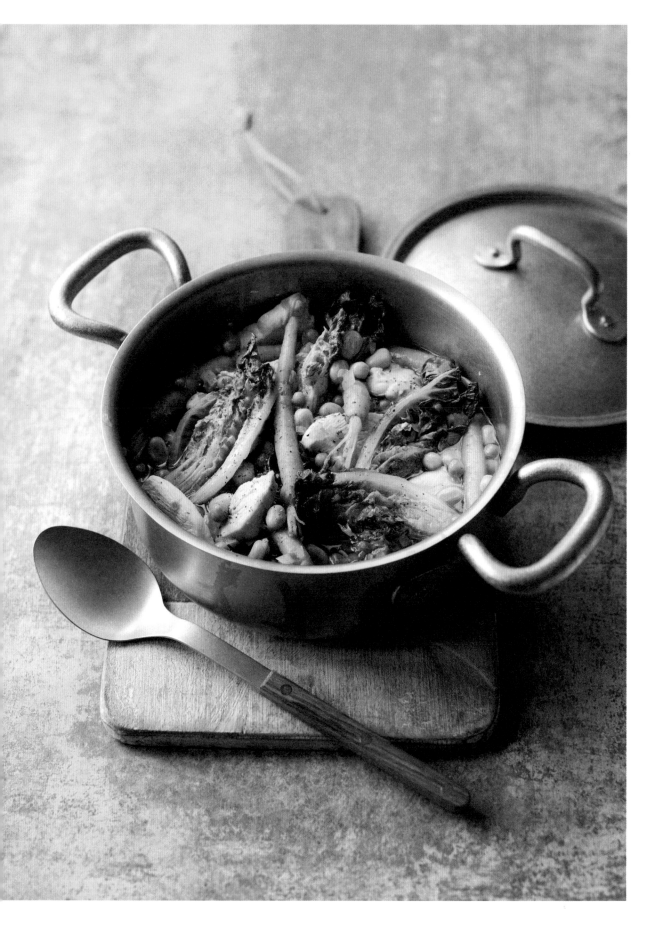

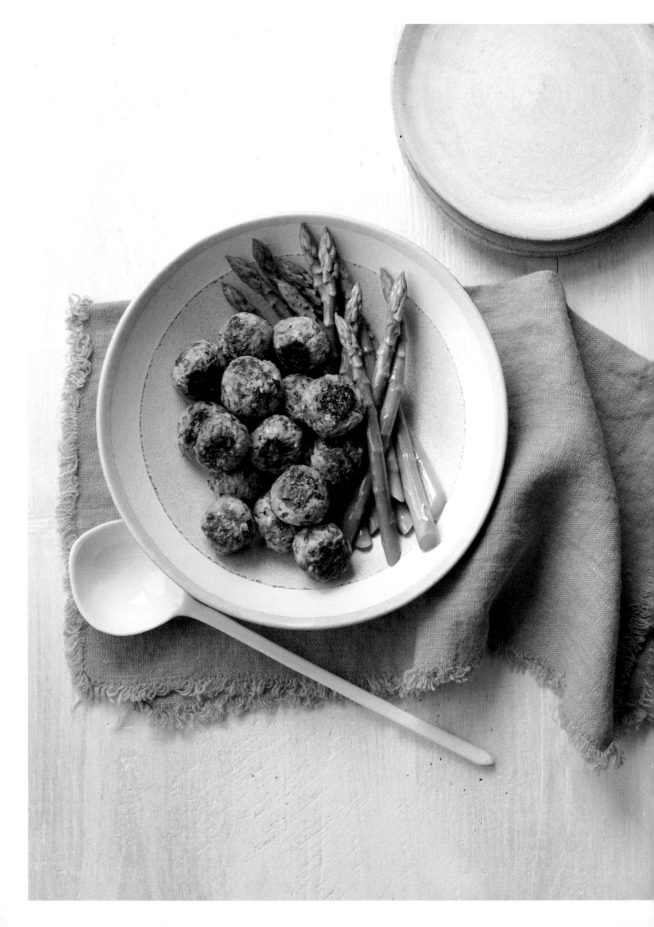

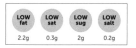

ENERGY 95kcals **PROTEIN** 12g | **FAT** 2.2g | **SATURATED FAT** 0.3g
CARBOHYDRATE 3g | **TOTAL SUGARS** 2g | **SALT** 0.2g | **SODIUM** 82mg | **FIBRE** 1g

Chicken Meatballs with Garlic, Herbs & Paprika

GF

If using gluten-free soy sauce

Nice easy recipe here and, yes, I do dry-fry the meatballs. You will find a certain amount of moisture is released from them as they cook, which helps to colour them. I don't ever fry paprika as it burns and tastes awful, so you should always add it to a mix or liquid. Be careful with the amount, as smoked paprika is very pungent and can overpower every other ingredient.

Serves 4

PREPARATION TIME: 25 minutes
COOKING TIME: 15 minutes

1 teaspoon rapeseed oil
2 small onions, very finely chopped
1 heaped tablespoon very finely chopped fresh ginger
1 garlic clove, crushed
200g chicken breast mince (skinless)
2 tablespoons chopped parsley
2 tablespoons chopped basil
2 tablespoons chopped chives
1 level tablespoon smoked paprika
1 teaspoon reduced-salt soy sauce
freshly ground black pepper

Heat the oil in a non-stick frying pan, then add the onions, ginger and garlic. Cook for 2–3 minutes to reduce some of their rawness. Set aside to cool.

Place the mince in a bowl and break up with a spatula, then add the herbs, paprika and cooled onion mix. Mix well and season with the soy sauce and pepper, then mix really well again. Roll into roughly 2.5cm balls, then chill really well for 3–4 minutes.

Gently heat a non-stick wok or frying pan over a medium heat. Add the meatballs and gently dry-fry for 8–10 minutes, rolling them around the pan to colour on all sides. Serve.

Cook's Tip
I serve these delicious meatballs with some steamed asparagus, pak choy or some lightly roasted cauliflower.

LOW fat	LOW sat	LOW sug	MED salt		ENERGY 269kcals **PROTEIN** 22g | **FAT** 1.2g | **SATURATED FAT** 0.3g
1.2g	0.3g	2.1g	0.5g		**CARBOHYDRATE** 42g | **TOTAL SUGARS** 2.1g | **SALT** 0.5g | **SODIUM** 196mg | **FIBRE** 4g

Fragrant Turkey Pho

GF

If using gluten-free stock cube

I was once very lucky to film in Vietnam some years ago. On every street corner in Hanoi they serve Pho from very early in the morning up until lunchtime. I had a beef version but the base stock was always the same, packed with fresh basil and lots of chilli. Pho is a very satisfying meal and is very good for you.

Serves 4

PREPARATION TIME: 30 minutes
COOKING TIME: 15 minutes

½ × 10g reduced-salt chicken stock cube
10 spring onions, sliced on the diagonal
1 small fresh red chilli, finely chopped
4 garlic cloves, crushed
1 teaspoon fish sauce
2 small skinless turkey breast slices (approx. 250g), fat trimmed
200g cooked rice vermicelli
200g beansprouts
6 tablespoons roughly chopped fresh coriander
4 tablespoons roughly chopped Thai or any fresh basil
10 fresh mint leaves, roughly chopped
juice of 2 large limes
freshly ground black pepper

Place 1 litre of water and the stock cube into a large saucepan and heat until just simmering.

Next add the onions, chilli, garlic, fish sauce and some pepper. Simmer for 3 minutes.

Cut the turkey into very thin slices and then add to the stock: it will cook almost straight away. Stir well.

Add the vermicelli noodles and beansprouts and bring back to a simmer, then turn off the heat.

Add the herbs to the Pho along with the juice from the lime and serve straight away.

Nutrition Tip

A leaner meat than chicken, turkey is a good source of B vitamins, selenium, zinc and phosphorus.

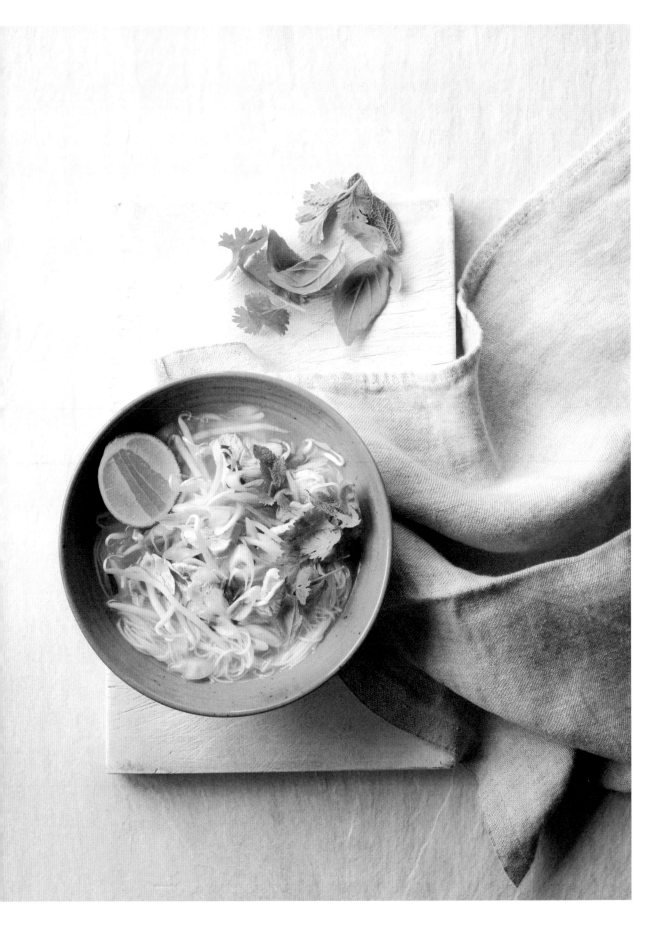

ENERGY 382kcals **PROTEIN** 39g | **FAT** 12g | **SATURATED FAT** 2.9g
CARBOHYDRATE 29g | **TOTAL SUGARS** 4g | **SALT** 0.5g | **SODIUM** 184mg | **FIBRE** 4g

Quick Pheasant & Lentil Curry

GF

If using gluten-free stock cube and asafoetida

This easy and very quick curry only takes a few minutes to cook. The sauce is thickened by breaking up the lentils, so just keep an eye on the liquid you add to get the right consistency. You can, of course, use a can of cooked lentils to make the dish even quicker to cook. I sometimes use this base for a vegetarian or vegan curry using cooked or canned pulses and vegetables and swapping the stock cube for a vegetable one.

Serves 4

PREPARATION TIME: 20 minutes
COOKING TIME: 30–40 minutes

FOR THE SPICE MIX
1 teaspoon rapeseed oil
1 tablespoon black mustard seeds
1 teaspoon ground turmeric
1 teaspoon ground cumin
1 tablespoon black onion seeds
1 teaspoon asafoetida

FOR THE CURRY
1 tablespoon finely chopped ginger
1 tablespoon chopped fresh red chilli
2 small onions, very finely chopped
2 garlic cloves, very finely chopped
175g red lentils
300ml boiling water
10g reduced-salt chicken stock cube
2 ripe tomatoes, chopped
3 tablespoons chopped fresh
   coriander
2 tablespoons chopped fresh mint

FOR THE PHEASANT
4 young pheasant breasts, skinned
   and deboned (approx. 120g each)
1 egg white, lightly broken up with
   a fork
freshly ground black pepper

Heat the oil in a non-stick saucepan over a medium heat, then add the spices and cook for 2–3 minutes to give them a little colour.

Next add the ginger, chilli, onions, garlic, lentils, boiling water and stock cube and bring to the boil.

Reduce the heat to a simmer and cook for 15–20 minutes until the lentils are cooked and just starting to break up. The sauce should be nice and thick now.

Cut the pheasant into 2–3cm pieces, dust with a little pepper and pop into the egg white, coating well. Drop the pheasant pieces into the lentil stew mix and stir well to set the egg white.

Simmer for 2–3 minutes, then remove the pan from the stove, add the tomatoes, cover and leave to rest for 15 minutes.

Once rested, stir well and check the seasoning. Add the herbs and stir through, then serve.

Cook's Tip

An unusual ingredient here is asafoetida with its deep savoury flavour profile: if you cannot eat onions or garlic, this is a good flavour replacer for those ingredients. If you can't find asafoetida, use 4–5 fresh or dried curry leaves.

Try swapping the pheasant for chicken of the same weight; give it a few more minutes to cook thoroughly.

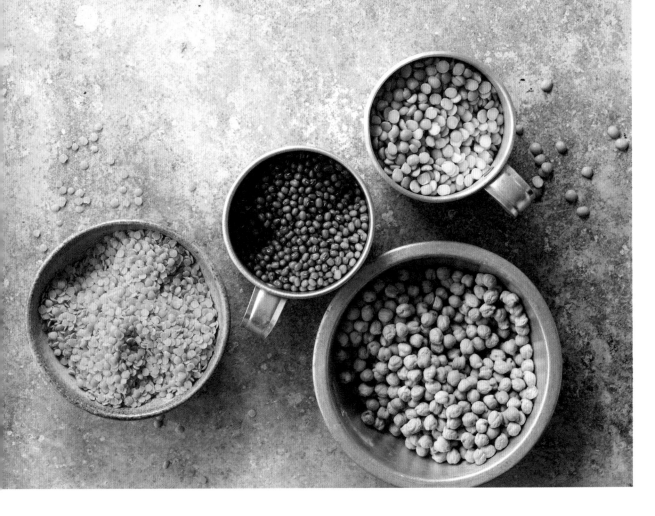

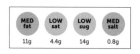

| MED fat 11g | LOW sat 4.4g | LOW sug 14g | MED salt 0.8g |

ENERGY 358kcals **PROTEIN** 13g | **FAT** 11g | **SATURATED FAT** 4.4g
CARBOHYDRATE 53g | **TOTAL SUGARS** 14g | **SALT** 0.8g | **SODIUM** 325mg | **FIBRE** 13g

Twice Baked Sweet Potatoes with Sausages & Beans

GF
If using gluten-free sausages

My mother used to cook us twice-baked jackets as a kid, and I've always liked them since. It turns a simple baked potato in a full main course. Pretty much anything goes and works really well. I sometimes microwave the potatoes for 4–5 minutes to start them cooking, cutting down the time spent in the oven to roughly half of what it would be otherwise.

Serves 4

PREPARATION TIME: 15 minutes
COOKING TIME: 1 hour

4 large sweet potatoes (600g)
4 low-fat chicken sausages (25–30g
 each), cut into small pieces
2 onions, finely chopped
2 garlic cloves, crushed
400g can kidney beans, drained
 well and rinsed
50g very finely grated Parmesan
 (optional)
freshly ground black pepper

Preheat the oven to 220°C/200°C fan/gas mark 7.

Wash the sweet potatoes well and place in the oven. Cook for 1 hour or until soft with crunchy skins.

Meanwhile, heat a non-stick sauté pan over a low heat. Add the sausages, onions and garlic and cook for 4–5 minutes to soften. Add the beans and warm through, then transfer to a bowl.

Remove the potatoes from the oven and halve lengthways, then spoon the hot potato into a bowl. You want to keep the skins intact, so leave a good 5mm or so of flesh on the skin.

Place the potato flesh into the bowl with the sausage, onion and beans, then mix well and add a little pepper. Spoon the mixture back into the shells, piling nice and high, then evenly sprinkle over the cheese, if using. Pop under a grill or in a hot oven to brown slightly for 5–6 minutes and serve.

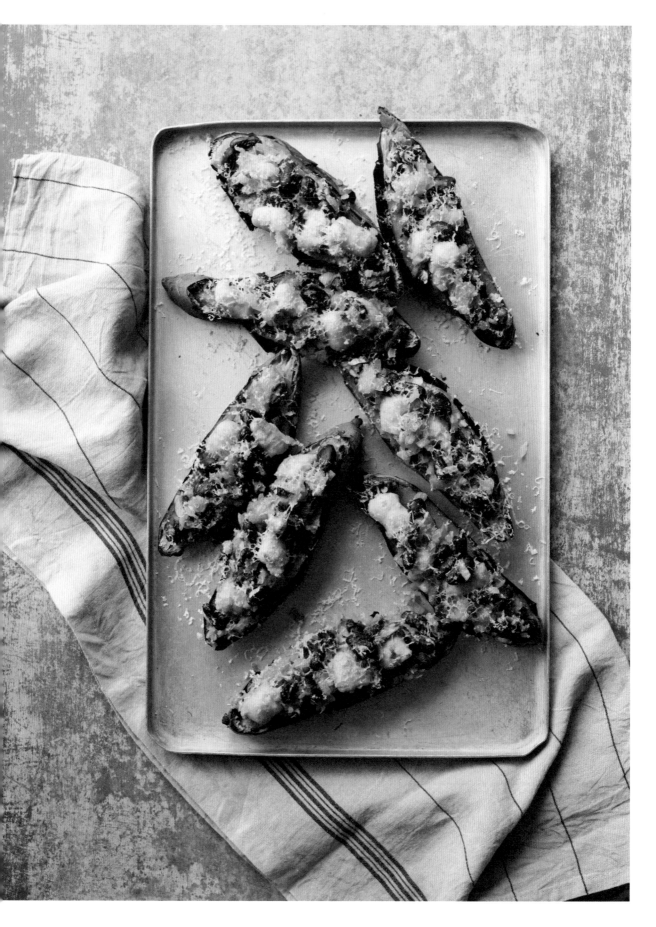

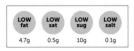

LOW fat	LOW sat	LOW sug	LOW salt
4.7g	0.5g	10g	0.1g

ENERGY 164kcals **PROTEIN** 21g | **FAT** 4.7g | **SATURATED FAT** 0.5g
CARBOHYDRATE 11g | **TOTAL SUGARS** 10g | **SALT** 0.1g | **SODIUM** 46mg | **FIBRE** 3.9g

Easy Spiced Turkey with Peppers & Tomatoes

I really like simple easy recipes and this is a typical one using that approach. Just simmer all the vegetables and spices, then sauté the turkey and add that's it. No browning: just pop it all in and get on with your life...

Serves 4

PREPARATION TIME: 30 minutes
COOKING TIME: 15 minutes

FOR THE STEW
1 small onion, very finely chopped
1 small red pepper, deseeded and sliced
1 small yellow pepper, deseeded and sliced
1 small green pepper, deseeded and sliced
2 tablespoons very finely chopped fresh ginger
2 garlic cloves, finely chopped
1–2 teaspoons roughly chopped fresh red chilli
1 level teaspoon ground cumin
1 level teaspoon ground coriander
½ teaspoon ground turmeric
1 tablespoon tomato purée
400g can chopped tomatoes

FOR THE TURKEY
1 tablespoon rapeseed oil
300g turkey breast, cut into 1cm strips
freshly ground black pepper
4 tablespoons chopped fresh coriander, to serve

Place all the ingredients for the stew into a pan, along with an extra 200ml of water swilled around the tomato can. Bring to the boil, then simmer for about 10 minutes or so until you have a thick stew.

Heat the oil in a non-stick wok or large frying pan, then add the turkey pieces and cook for 4–5 minutes until well browned and cooked through: do not overcook.

Place the cooked turkey into the stew and cook for a further 2–3 minutes. Finally season with a little pepper and add lots of coriander. Serve with wholegrain basmati rice, if you like.

Nutrition Tip
Red are the most nutritious of the bell peppers as they are left on the vine longest. They have 11 times more beta-carotene and 1.5 times more vitamin C than green peppers, which are picked first, before they have a chance to turn yellow, orange and then red.

| LOW fat 1.9g | LOW sat 0.8g | LOW sug 6.5g | MED salt 0.4g |

ENERGY 151kcals **PROTEIN** 26g | **FAT** 1.9g | **SATURATED FAT** 0.8g
CARBOHYDRATE 8.3g | **TOTAL SUGARS** 6.5g | **SALT** 0.4g | **SODIUM** 200mg | **FIBRE** 3g

Venison meatloaf

GF

I really like meatloaf in any form: here is a venison version
that is really tasty, though you can try it with reduced-fat
minced beef, too. I have purposely cut down the meat to
100g per person and bulked it out with mushrooms to keep
volume to the dish. You can eat this warm straight from the
oven or leave it to cool, then chill in the fridge and eat cold
like you would a pâté. You may think it's slightly unusual to
see this kind of recipe, but do give it a try.

Serves 4

PREPARATION TIME: 20 minutes
COOKING TIME: 1 hour

250g brown mushrooms, finely
    chopped
4 onions, finely chopped
4 garlic cloves, finely chopped
400g 0%-fat minced venison
2 teaspoons dried oregano
1 teaspoon ground cinnamon
1 teaspoon dried chilli flakes
1 teaspoon allspice
1 egg white
4 tablespoons roughly chopped
    parsley
freshly ground black pepper

Preheat the oven to 180°C/160°C fan/gas mark 4.

Place the mushrooms, onions and garlic into a non-stick frying pan
over a medium heat and fry for 10 minutes to drive off all the moisture
that will come out of the onions and mushrooms.

Next spoon the mixture into a bowl and leave to cool slightly. Add the
venison, oregano, spices, egg white, parsley and pepper and mix really
well. Spoon into a small, 20cm square, 10cm deep baking dish and cover
tightly with foil. Place onto a baking tray and pop into the oven. Cook
for 35–45 minutes, or until the juices run clear once a knife is inserted.

Once cooked, carefully remove from the oven and leave to cool. Pop
into the fridge and chill well, best overnight.

Remove from the baking dish, then slice and wrap in clean foil or
clingfilm. Keep in the fridge until ready to use. This can be reheated,
sliced, in a microwave set to medium power, or eaten cold with salad.

Nutrition Tip
When mushrooms are exposed to sunlight (UV) it increases their
concentration of vitamin D. Try putting them on the windowsill for a
couple of hours, gills up, to boost the vitamin content.

Blueprint Burgers

If only a burger will do, it is possible to keep it on the healthy side. Fake-away the right bun, burger and everything in-between. Serve it with oven-baked sweet potato chips; very easy to make yourself.

The bun: Make it smaller and thinner. Choose a wholemeal bun; if it's seeded, even better.

The burger: Swap the beef in the burger for a leaner source of protein like grilled chicken or fish. Try the Spiced Fish Cakes on page 120.

Alternatively, go for plant protein: make your own veggie burger and load it high with contrasting textures and flavours. Try the recipe for Beetroot and Feta Falafels (page 85); the mixture will easily shape into a burger for your bun. Or try the vegan Aubergine and Bean Burgers on page 91.

The fillings: Opt for healthy toppers to add crunch, like a classic coleslaw. Try my Fennel Slaw Salad recipe on page 68; it's lighter than the mayonnaise version. Then there's the obvious crispy lettuce and fresh tomato. Plus you can go for reduced-fat cheese options, if you are trying to lose weight.

The toppers: Burgers need a spread to compliment the filling, but don't sabotage yourself with saturated fat and calories in the mayo dressing and sauces. You can add loads of flavour with herbs, spring onions and a creamy sliver of avocado, tangy mustard and chilli sauce; you will likely use much less of these. A few drops of chipotle chilli sauce in a spoon of unsweetened Greek-style yogurt will punch a hot smoky flavour into a small amount of dressing, which you can spread on your burger.

For more ideas, see the recipes for Hot Red Pepper Dressing, Herb & Tofu Green Dressing and Avocado & Herb Dressing (see opposite and pages 77 and 76).

Loaded burger: Halve the bun, place your choice of hot burger inside, drizzle the dressing over the burger and stack with the veggie layers. Serve with a small portion of Sweet Potato Fries (see page 71).

LOW fat 1.6g	LOW sat 0.8g	LOW sug 1g	LOW salt 0.25g

ENERGY 32kcals **PROTEIN** 2.4g | **FAT** 1.6g | **SATURATED FAT** 0.8g
CARBOHYDRATE 2g | **TOTAL SUGARS** 1g | **SALT** 0.25g | **SODIUM** 123mg | **FIBRE** 0.5g

Hot Red Pepper Dressing

Serves 4

100g roasted red pepper, finely chopped
4 tablespoons 0%-fat unsweetened Greek-style yogurt
small sliver of garlic (optional)
1 teaspoon lime or lemon juice, to taste
a sprinkling of dried chilli flakes or Tabasco (optional)

Put all the ingredients into a small food-processor (or use a stick blender) and process to a smooth, creamy dressing.

Add a cautious few drops of tabasco or a sprinkling of chilli flakes for a hot sauce version.

Nutrition Tip
Peppers are packed with nutrition, particularly red peppers, which are good sources of beta-carotene and vitamin C.

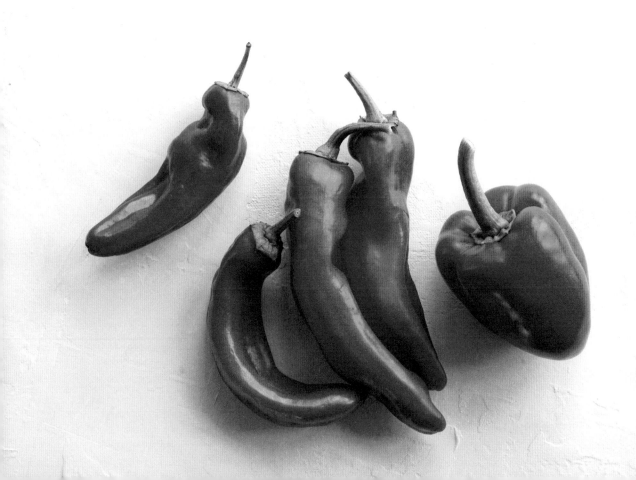

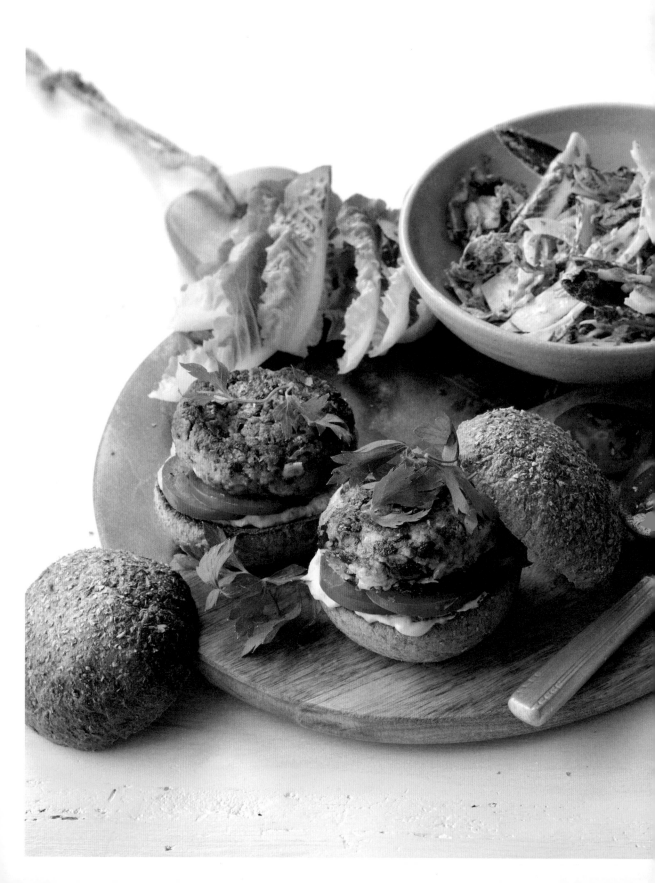

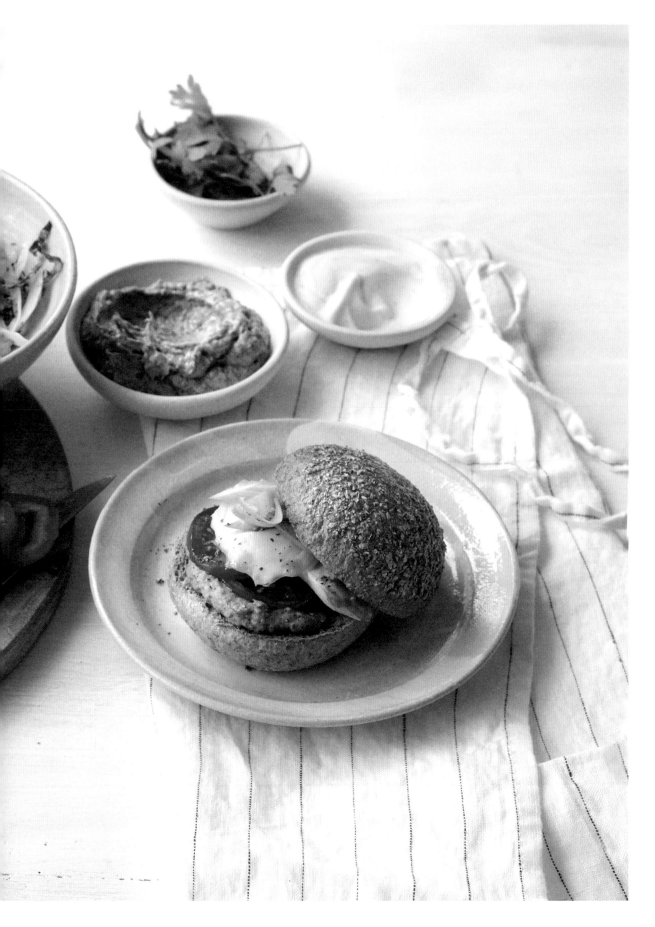

Sweets
& Treats

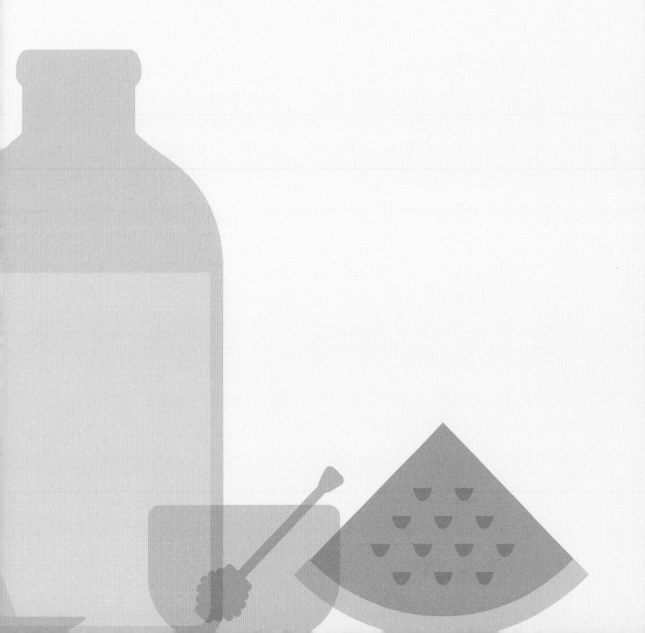

MED fat	MED sat	MED sug	MED salt
5g	1.4g	8.3g	0.1g

ENERGY 145kcals **PROTEIN** 4.3g | **FAT** 5g | **SATURATED FAT** 1.4g
CARBOHYDRATE 39g | **TOTAL SUGARS** 8.3g | **SALT** 0.1g | **SODIUM** 29mg | **FIBRE** 2.6g

Banana, Oat & Peanut Cookie Balls

If using gluten-free oats

Three simple ingredients make a soft, cookie-style portion, for when you want something to nibble. No added sugar here: the bananas provide all the sweetness needed and you get the benefit of fibre from the oats and healthy nut protein. These soft cookies are good to take with you for a snack. Keep the rest in the fridge for a few days or freeze and use within 2 months.

Makes 6

PREPARATION TIME: 10 minutes
COOKING TIME: 15–20 minutes

2 medium, ripe bananas, peeled (200g peeled weight)
100g porridge oats
50g crunchy peanut butter

Preheat the oven to 180°C/160°C fan/gas mark 4. Line a baking tray with a sheet of greaseproof paper.

Mash the bananas with a fork in a bowl, until mostly smooth. Add the oats and the peanut butter. Mix well to combine into a soft dough.

Portion the mixture in to six, about 1 heaped tablespoon each, and flatten into rough rounds on the greaseproof paper. Bake in a hot oven until just firm: about 15–20 minutes.

Allow to cool. The rounds will remain soft but not sticky and make conveniently small portions.

Nutrition Tip

The soluble type of fibre found in oats (beta-glucan) can help to lower cholesterol and is associated with a reduced risk of heart disease.

Note

The sugar in this recipe and the recipe opposite comes from fruit or dried fruit and the majority of fat is from healthier sources such as nuts, seeds, oats and dairy. These recipes provide a healthier snack alternative compared to many commercially available snacks. As ever it's important to be mindful of portion size.

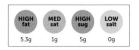

HIGH fat	MED sat	HIGH sug	LOW salt
5.3g	1g	5g	0g

ENERGY 100kcals **PROTEIN** 3.2g | **FAT** 5.3g | **SATURATED FAT** 1g
CARBOHYDRATE 10g | **TOTAL SUGARS** 5g | **SALT** 0g | **SODIUM** 0mg | **FIBRE** 2g

Chocolate Power Balls

If using gluten-free oats

A nutritious energy boost in a snack-sized bite. Make some of these for when you fancy something sweet and only chocolate will hit the spot: these snacks are chocolatey and I like to use dates to bind it all together, as a source of natural sugar and fibre.

Makes 4

PREPARATION TIME: 10 minutes

25g pitted soft dates
2 tablespoons boiling water
1 tablespoon (10g) cocoa powder, unsweetened
1 tablespoon (10g) ground super seeds mix (see tip)
1 tablespoon (10g) ground almonds
2 tablespoons jumbo oats

Chop the dates finely. Place in a small bowl with the boiling water and mash to a soft pulp using a fork. Medjool dates will need less water, other dates may need the full 2 tablespoons: if they are really dry, then pop them in the microwave for 30 seconds and then mash them.

Slowly mix in all the other ingredients and work the paste together. It might seem too stiff at first but keep going: it will form a thick paste, which you can then roll it into four balls. If you aren't going to eat them now, wrap in clingfilm and pop them in the fridge for later. These snacks will happily keep in an airtight container in the fridge for a couple of days but will become drier, as the flaxseeds absorb a lot of moisture.

Cook's Tip

Look for a blend of ground super seeds in a pre-mixed pack, such as milled golden flaxseeds with sunflower, pumpkin and sesame seeds: packs are available in supermarkets.

Try adding 1 teaspoon of dried fruit, such as sour cherries, or some grated fresh ginger for a different flavour.

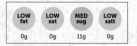

LOW fat	LOW sat	MED sug	LOW salt
0g	0g	11g	0g

ENERGY 45kcals | **PROTEIN** 1g | **FAT** 0g | **SATURATED FAT** 0g
CARBOHYDRATE 11g | **TOTAL SUGARS** 11g | **SALT** 0g | **SODIUM** 0mg | **FIBRE** 2.7g

Plum Compote

Ve

GF

Plums, I think, are underrated, yet they have plenty of the
good stuff; polyphenols and phytonutrients, especially the
red and purple varieties. The antioxidants are concentrated
in the skins, so leave these on when you cook them.
Roasting intensifies the natural sweetness in the fruit.

Serves 2

PREPARATION TIME: 5 minutes
COOKING TIME: 15 minutes

4 ripe plums, halved and stoned

Preheat the oven to 200°C/180°C fan/gas mark 6.

Arrange the plums, cut side up, in a shallow baking dish lined with
greaseproof paper. Spoon over 1 tablespoon of water. Bake in a hot
oven for about 15 minutes, until soft.

Cook's Tip

This soft compote of plums is delicious to add to sweet and savoury
dishes. For breakfast, serve with kefir cultures in a high-protein yogurt
or any other type of unsweetened yogurt. Top with a sprinkling of
chopped raw almonds, skin on. For a salad, leave out the water and
roast the fruit dry: add to green salad with sugar snap peas, rocket
and watercress and a matchbox-sized portion of feta.

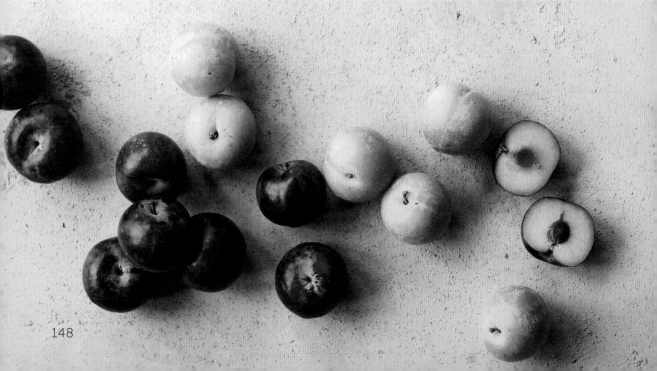

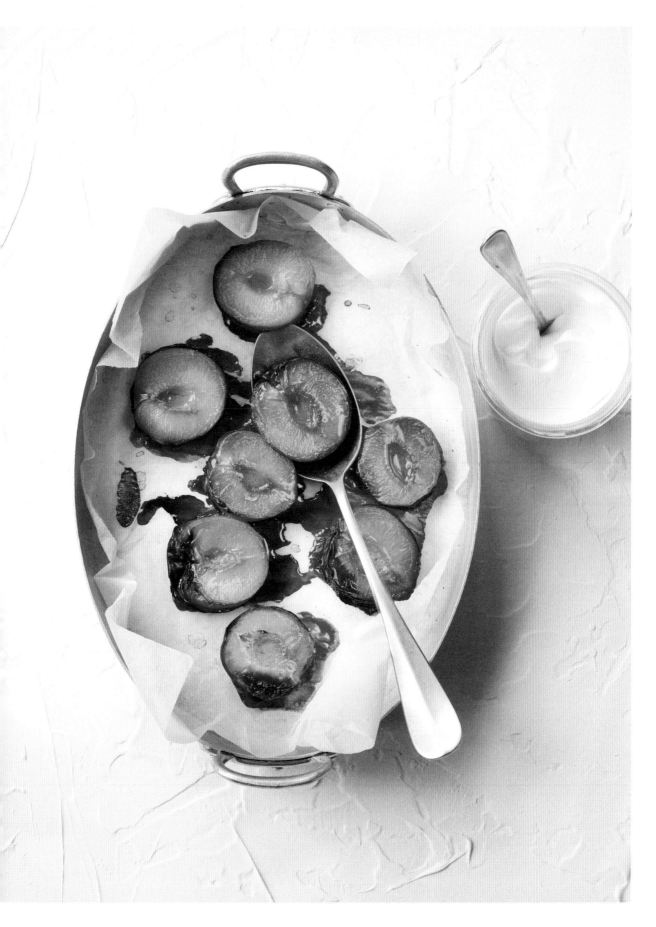

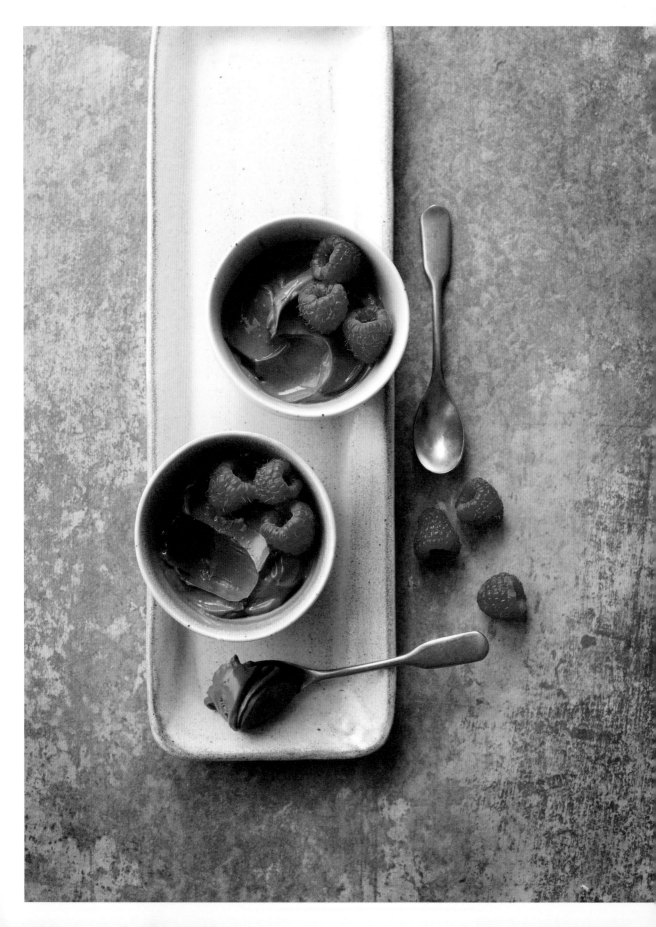

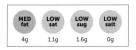

ENERGY 75kcals **PROTEIN** 6.3g | **FAT** 4g | **SATURATED FAT** 1.1g
CARBOHYDRATE 3.7g | **TOTAL SUGARS** 1.6g | **SALT** 0g | **SODIUM** 0mg | **FIBRE** 1g

Silky Chocolate Mousse

If using
vegan dark
chocolate

Silken tofu is creamy and smooth with a subtle flavour that lends itself to thicken and create this chocolatey treat. It just happens to be vegan and low calorie, too.

Serves 2

PREPARATION TIME: 10 minutes

150g silken tofu, drained
2½ teaspoons vanilla extract
1 tablespoon unsweetened cocoa
    powder
5g dark chocolate

Pat dry the tofu and then purée in a food-processor or blender for a few seconds until smooth.

Add the vanilla, sift in the cocoa (to avoid lumps) and blend briefly.

Melt the chocolate on low power in a microwave until runny. (If the chocolate cools too fast the texture might become grainy instead of mixing in smoothly.) Add to the tofu mixture in the food-processor. Pulse until smooth.

Divide between two little serving dishes, such as ramekins, and pop in the fridge to chill until ready to serve.

Nutrition Tips

Serving with a few cherries or raspberries on the side will add some useful fibre.

Dark chocolate with a high cocoa content (70% or more) is a good source of iron, magnesium, copper, manganese, potassium, phosphorus, zinc and selenium.

| MED fat 3.4g | MED sat 1.2g | LOW sug 1.8g | MED salt 0.8g |

ENERGY 156kcals **PROTEIN** 8.1g | **FAT** 3.4g | **SATURATED FAT** 1.2g

CARBOHYDRATE 25g | **TOTAL SUGARS** 1.8g | **SALT** 0.8g | **SODIUM** 324mg | **FIBRE** 3.8g

Bitter Chocolate Muffins

This is a nice, simple recipe: just mix the wet and dry ingredients together and bake off! However, do not overmix when combining the ingredients or the cooked muffins will be tough and chewy.

Makes 8

PREPARATION TIME: 15 minutes
COOKING TIME: 15 minutes

FOR THE DRY
35g cocoa powder
2 level teaspoons baking powder
1 teaspoon bicarbonate of soda
250g wholemeal flour

FOR THE WET
2 medium eggs
1 teaspoon vanilla extract
3 tablespoons granulated
   sweetener
200ml skimmed milk

Preheat the oven to 180°C /160°C fan/gas mark 4.

In a bowl, mix together the cocoa, baking powder, bicarb and wholemeal flour really well.

In a separate bowl, combine the eggs, vanilla, sweetener and milk, and mix well. Add this egg mixture to the dry bowl and mix very lightly (see above).

Spoon into the muffin cases and pop into the oven. Bake for 15–20 minutes: do not overcook or the muffins will be dry.

Once well risen and soft to the touch, remove from the oven and cool.

Note
The majority of fat in this recipe is from healthier sources such as eggs and dairy. This recipe provides a healthier snack alternative compared to many commercially available snacks. As ever it's important to be mindful of portion size.

				ENERGY 93kcals	PROTEIN 9.1g	FAT 1.7g	SATURATED FAT 0.8g
LOW fat	LOW sat	MED sug	LOW salt	CARBOHYDRATE 11g	TOTAL SUGARS 11g	SALT 0g	SODIUM 169mg	FIBRE 3.8g
1.7g	0.8g	11g	0g				

Strawberries on Sweet Cottage Cheese

GF

Celebrate the strawberry season with a new taste for breakfast: try it!

Serves 1

7 strawberries (100g), sliced
2 tablespoons low-fat cottage
    cheese
½ teaspoon honey

Just pile the strawberries into a bowl and top with the cottage cheese and honey drizzle.

Nutrition Tip

This is incredibly simple for a snack, or something sweet, and provides nutritious protein, fibre and vitamins. Strawberries are also low calorie, packed with antioxidants and rich in vitamin C.

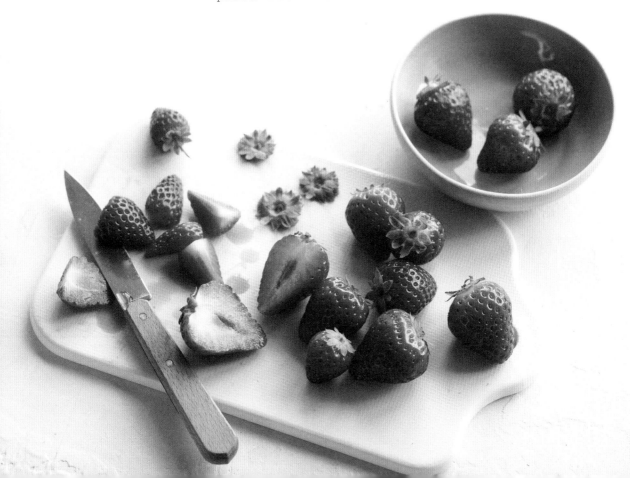

LOW fat 3g	LOW sat 1.2g	MED sug 11g	LOW salt 0g	**ENERGY** 109kcals **PROTEIN** 5.6g | **FAT** 3g | **SATURATED FAT** 1.2g
				CARBOHYDRATE 14g | **TOTAL SUGARS** 11g | **SALT** 0g | **SODIUM** 0mg | **FIBRE** 1g

Watermelon with Saffron Yogurt Basil & Mint

I really like this serving method for any watermelon dish, sweet or savoury. Hand on heart, I saw the idea when I filmed in the Turks & Caicos Islands, where chef Colin Watson at Sandals Beach reigns supreme.

Serves 4

PREPARATION TIME: 20 minutes

a few saffron stamens
2 tablespoons boiling water
3cm-thick slice watermelon
150g 0%-fat unsweetened yogurt
10 fresh mint leaves
10 fresh basil leaves (I prefer Thai basil)
2 tablespoons sunflower seeds, lightly toasted
freshly ground black pepper (optional)

Place the saffron into an egg cup and add the boiling water. Stir and then leave to cool.

Place the watermelon slice onto a large serving plate and remove any seeds with a fork, then cut into eight even wedges.

Beat the yogurt and then spread evenly over the melon, leaving 2cm at the edge; it's nice to see the colour contrast, especially when you add more ingredients.

Finely slice the mint and basil and sprinkle over the yogurt, then add the toasted seeds.

Just before serving, spoon over the lovely saffron water and a little black pepper, if using. Serve straight away.

Nutrition Tip
Watermelon is one of the best fruits to eat if you're trying to lose weight since 90% of its weight is water and, as a result, it is low in calories.

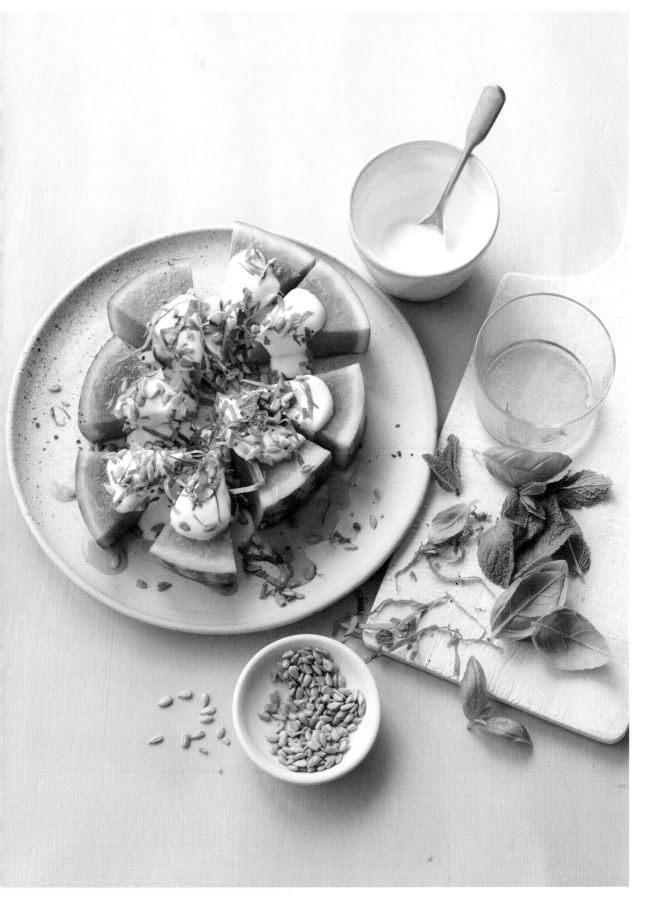

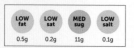

ENERGY 70kcals **PROTEIN** 5.6g | **FAT** 0.5g | **SATURATED FAT** 0.2g
CARBOHYDRATE 12g | **TOTAL SUGARS** 11g | **SALT** 0.1g | **SODIUM** 67mg | **FIBRE** 0.6g

LOW fat	LOW sat	MED sug	LOW salt
0.5g	0.2g	11g	0.1g

Pannacotta

Really easy recipe here: just remember to soak the leaf gelatine first for 10 minutes in cold water. This ensures that it will immediately dissolve once added to the hot milk. I serve this with a few berries scattered over. I also like frozen blueberries and blackcurrants, as they tend to extrude a lovely juice when defrosted.

Serves 4

PREPARATION TIME: 15 minutes
COOKING TIME: 10 minutes

600ml skimmed milk
4 gelatine leaves, soaked in cold water until soft
1 level tablespoon granulated sweetener
1 teaspoon rose or orange flower water
150g fresh or frozen blueberries (defrosted)

Place the milk into a saucepan and bring to a simmer. Once simmering remove from the heat and leave to cool for 10 minutes.

Once slightly cooled, squeeze the excess water from the gelatine, then stir into the milk with the sweetener and rose or orange flower water. Stir well until dissolved.

Pour evenly into four medium-sized ramekins, then place in a fridge to set, probably best overnight. Once chilled, they will still be slightly wobbly in the centre.

When ready to serve, run a knife around the edge of the set milk. Dip the base of the ramekin in a bowl of hot water for 15–20 seconds, then carefully turn out onto a plate or bowl. Serve with a few berries dotted around and over.

Cook's Tip
Ensure you add the sweetener once the milk has cooled for a few minutes, as some sweeteners are not very heat stable and you can lose sweetness if they become hot.

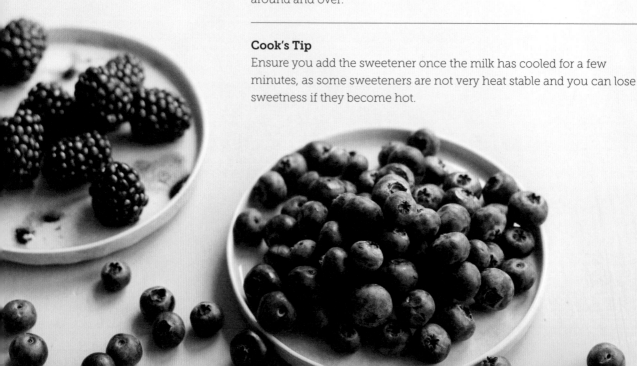

LOW fat	LOW sat	LOW sug	LOW salt
4.5g	1.3g	7.3g	0.2g

ENERGY 139kcals **PROTEIN** 13g | **FAT** 4.5g | **SATURATED FAT** 1.3g

CARBOHYDRATE 12g | **TOTAL SUGARS** 7.3g | **SALT** 0.2g | **SODIUM** 141mg | **FIBRE** 0.5g

Vanilla Blancmange

Some years ago, I won chef of the year with this blancmange recipe as my dessert, albeit with conventional sugar. So I thought I'd create a sugar-free version, and I have to say, it works really well if you fancy a light dessert and serve with a little fresh fruit.

Serves 4

PREPARATION TIME: 20 minutes
COOKING TIME: 10 minutes

3 eggs
300ml skimmed milk
1 tablespoon custard powder
2 teaspoons vanilla extract
4 gelatine leaves, soaked in cold
    water until soft
1 tablespoon granulated sweetener
300g fat-free fromage frais

Separate the eggs, ensuring there are no traces of yolk in the whites. Lightly beat the egg white and set aside for later.

Gently heat the milk and vanilla in a small pan.

In a small bowl, mix the custard powder with 2 tablespoons of cold water. Once the milk is just simmering, whisk in the custard mixture. Cook until thickened very slightly, then remove from the heat and leave to cool for 5 minutes.

Once cooled, whisk the custard mixture into the egg yolks. Return to the pan and cook over a gentle heat until the custard thickens slightly, then remove from the heat and add the softened gelatine and the sweetener.

Place into a clean bowl and sit the bowl over some ice cubes. Stir occasionally until the mixture starts to thicken slightly. This part is really important: if the mix is not chilled and thickened enough to hold its own weight, the mix will not set evenly and will split.

Next quickly whisk in the fromage frais and finally the lightly beaten egg white.

Spoon into four small dishes or a large bowl and chill until set. Serve with a few raspberries on top.

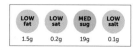

ENERGY 188kcals **PROTEIN** 4g | **FAT** 1.5g | **SATURATED FAT** 0.2g
CARBOHYDRATE 42g | **TOTAL SUGARS** 19g | **SALT** 0.1g | **SODIUM** 131mg | **FIBRE** 2.7g

Banana Spring Rolls

Ve
If using
vegan filo

A nice and simple recipe that is packed with flavour and really easy to make. I sometimes freeze these first and bake from frozen; just allow an extra 15–20 minutes on the cooking time.

Serves 4

PREPARATION TIME: 20 minutes
COOKING TIME: 12–15 minutes

4 sheets filo pastry
2–3 sprays of rapeseed oil
4 small ripe bananas, peeled
1 level teaspoon ground allspice
small bunch of Thai basil, finely
   chopped

Preheat the oven to 200°C/180°C fan/gas mark 6.

Lay out the four sheets of filo pastry, then spray lightly with oil. Place a banana on one end of each pastry sheet, then sprinkle with a little allspice and chopped basil. Roll the pastry over to cover the banana, then tuck in the sides. Finish by rolling up nice and tightly.

Place on a non-stick baking sheet and spray again lightly. Bake in the oven for 12–15 minutes.

Leave to cool for 10 minutes before eating.

Nutrition Tip
Bananas are high in fibre and contain rich amounts of potassium, which may help reduce blood pressure and water retention and also protect against stroke.

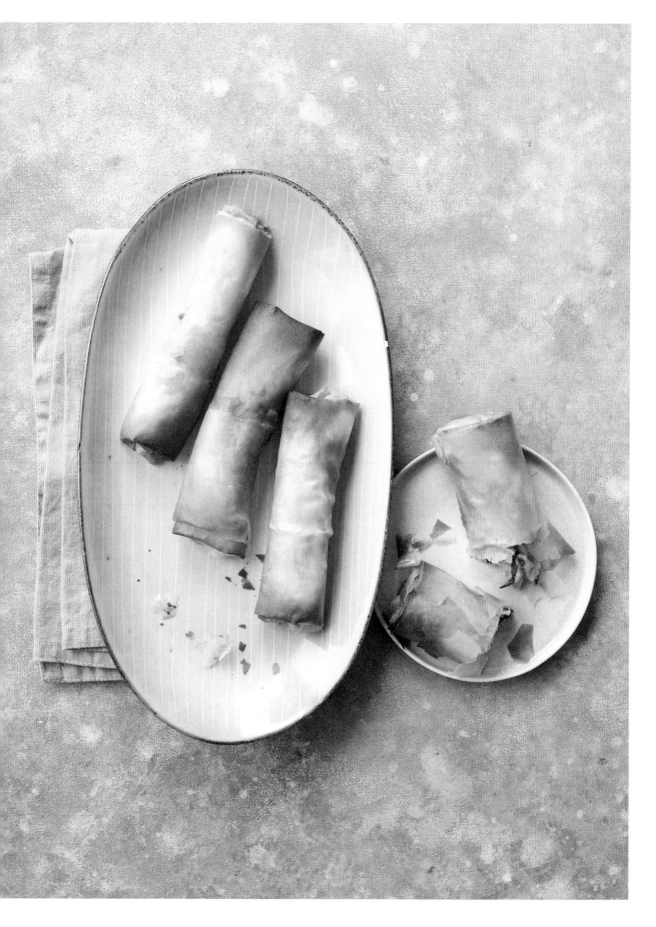

Meal Planners

8

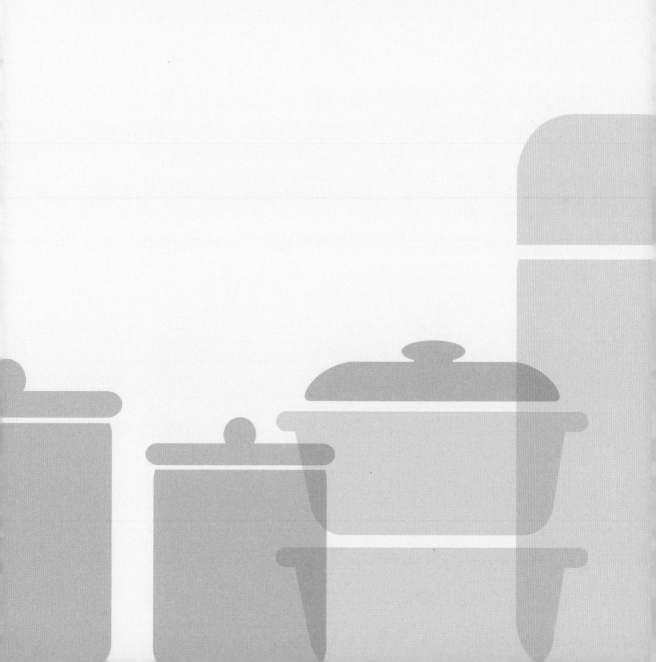

Weight Loss and Diabetes

There are so many benefits to losing extra weight – both physically and emotionally. It could help the insulin you produce or inject work better by reducing insulin resistance. You may be able to reduce the dose of your diabetes medication, along with your healthcare team. It will help you reduce the risk of long-term complications. Although getting Type 1 diabetes has nothing to do with weight, losing any extra weight still has benefits. And if you have Type 2 diabetes, there is strong evidence that losing extra weight can help to manage the condition better.

Type 2 Diabetes and Weight Loss

Extra weight around your waist means fat can build up around organs, like your liver and pancreas. This can cause something called insulin resistance and means your body can't use insulin properly, increasing your chances of high blood glucose levels and type 2 diabetes. Especially if you are newly diagnosed, overweight or obese, scientists believe that you will stand a good chance of putting type 2 diabetes into remission if you lose weight (around 10–15kg is significant, although losing even a little will mean better health). There is no easy answer to achieving a remission – or guarantee it won't return – as diabetes is complex, but considering what we know so far, there are good indications that making changes to diet and lifestyle can be a game changer*.

*A clinical trial carried out at Newcastle University (DiRECT) suggested that a low-calorie diet (around 850 calories a day, under strict medical supervision) could put some people with type 2 diabetes into remission. More detail is needed: further research into low-calorie eating is being funded by Diabetes UK and currently being investigated by NHS England and Scotland.

Losing Weight

Everyone is different and there are many ways to tackle losing weight, so the best way is to find an approach that you can stick to and works for you. Importantly, ask the advice of your GP or dietician before starting any diet: you'll benefit from the support, and trying this without medical guidance could be dangerous if you use medications. Check the helpful guide to losing weight at www.diabetes.org.uk.

Remember, you need a good balance over the day from all the different food groups. If you plan to lose weight, you will aim to eat fewer calories than you need, so cut your default portion sizes and add more vegetables to fill your plate.

Regardless of whether you are aiming to lose weight or you are aiming to maintain weight, make it your goal to divide up the total calorie count throughout the day.

Planner to Lose Weight

All the meals in the planner are suggestions to include in a plan for losing weight, providing you stick to strict, smaller portion sizes. Low-calorie diets are not intended for the long term, may not be suitable for everyone and you may need a vitamin and mineral supplement. If you are taking certain types of diabetes medication always speak to your GP before starting a low-calorie diet. If you do not need to lose weight, or you are preparing meals for others who do not need to follow a strict diet, you can use these meal plans as a basis, then add extra healthy meals, sides and/or snacks: use the suggestions on the following pages for inspiration.

The secret to following a plan is to ensure that the food is really tasty while not using huge amounts of sugar, salt, fat or oil. This can be done with clever use of not only a strong and varied base ingredient, such as mushrooms, beans or noodles, but also herbs, spices and acidic flavours to get a well-balanced end result. See the top tips on page 13.

To lose weight, the average woman needs approximately 1,200 to 1,500 calories per day and the average man approximately 1,500 to 1,800 per day, though this obviously varies according to the individual and to activity levels. To lose weight, we suggest aiming to consume 600 fewer calories than you need per day, but always take advice from a dietician or doctor before you start.

When following a reduced-calorie diet, remember to:

- Aim for a good balance over the day from different food groups

- Target five-a-day fruit and veg

- Ensure you include two portions of oily fish during the week

- Eat sufficient fibre and whole grains

- Reduce your consumption of meat

- Watch out for hidden sources of fat, salt and sugar

Breakfast suggestions

Porridge
Always a good way to start the day, however, use water or skimmed milk to reduce calories. Adding fresh fruit will help to keep you fuller and hence fight off any urges later on.

Omelettes
Add a spoonful of drained, canned black beans to fill you up and add fibre and colour.

Yogurt and fruit
Chia yogurt and fruit: mix together and leave to chill overnight with some oats and a handful of fresh, or even frozen, raspberries or blueberries.

Eggs
Boiled, poached or scrambled on wholemeal toast, or even rice cakes, with a little avocado or mashed roasted sweet potato are good options.

Cereal
Reduced-salt wholegrain cereals are okay provided you stick to portion size and use skimmed milk.

Other breakfast ideas:

- Wafer-thin ham, turkey, etc. are really good mixed through scrambled eggs or served with courgette strips quickly fried in a non-stick pan with a dash of lemon juice.

- Drop scones made with wholemeal flour, egg, skimmed milk and seeded mustard are easy to make and great with a variety of toppings such as avocado, grilled sweet tomatoes, poached eggs and even a little wafer-thin ham.

- Vegetables such as courgette, pepper, aubergine, etc. roasted with a nice spice rub go well with a little tomato paste, topped with Greek yogurt; I really like this.

- Chickpea flour, canned chickpea and fresh ripe tomato pancakes are a light alternative, which you can make using no egg; bulk them out with fresh herbs such as parsley, coriander and tarragon.

- Thin egg omelettes: thin out with a little skimmed milk or water, cook, then roll up with fresh spinach and feta cheese – a perfect way to start the day.

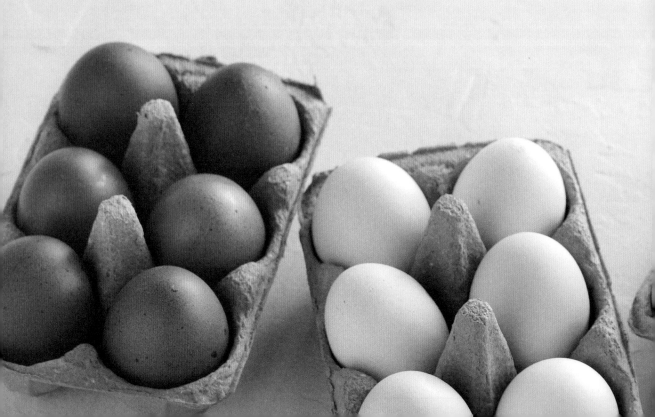

Lunch offerings

Bread
Use one or two slices of wholemeal bread with a thin layer of reduced-fat spread (on only one slice).

Dinner for lunch
Some main courses can double up as lunch and dinner offerings, such as Vegetable Scramble, Roasted Cauliflower Steaks and Five-pulse Jewelled Dal (see pages 80, 95 and 100). Omelettes are good to eat cold for lunch on-the-go.

Soup
Soups can be made in bulk and used for the next 2–3 days, either chilled or frozen and then microwaved to order. Cold gazpacho, tuna cauliflower broth and sweet potato vichyssoise are good and can be made in bulk.

Plan ahead
A lot of lunches can be made the night before, plus there are some very good microwavable sachets these days great for a busy day. These include quinoa, wild rice and mixed beans. They come in 250g sachets, and half a packet makes a great base for many tasty lunches or snacks.

Pasta
Small amounts of wholemeal pastas cooked and chilled then served cold or reheated, are a good way to sustain you for longer. Try wholewheat pasta (or gluten-free pasta made from lentils, pea protein, etc.), cooked and cooled. Eating the pasta cold or reheated makes the starchy carbs more resistant and slower to digest.

Other lunch ideas:
- Poached chicken (skinned) with spinach and black pepper.

- Smoked mackerel with a dash of hot horseradish.

- Baked potato or vegetable crisps rather than fried versions.

- Mix roasted veg with cold pasta, or reheat a small portion of wholegrain pasta with roasted vegetables and chopped tomatoes.

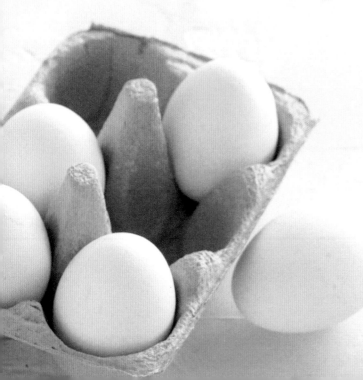

Suggestions for lunch on-the-go

Oily fish
Any oily fish are good in small amounts: they can be mixed with canned pulses, salad leaves and a touch of acid, such as vinegar or lemon or lime juice, to make a great healthy lunch; this can be made the night before.

Boiled eggs
Either soft- or hard-boiled, eggs are also really good. I often add them to cooked pulses or grains, or even a jar of roasted peppers or artichokes.

Fresh tuna
Seared rare, this can be a tasty treat, with a little crisp Romaine or little gem lettuce, a few sesame seeds, some black pepper and roasted garlic. Use small frozen portions of tuna, which are sold in all major supermarkets.

Rice noodles
Try ready-to-eat rice noodles: just add boiling water when you're ready to eat, and add a little fresh ginger, spring onions and a few spinach leaves; liven it all up with a splash of olive oil and cider vinegar, if you like.

Soups
Simple easy soups can be made from any veg left over: just simmer until soft, then either purée or leave chunky. Keep it hot in a flask or microwave at work for a healthy, filling lunchtime snack.

Rice
Wild rice microwave sachets are great and heat up in 2 minutes. Add simple flavourings such as fresh Thai or conventional basil, along with some fresh garlic, black pepper and a sprinkling of curry powder or garam masala to season for a tasty alternative.

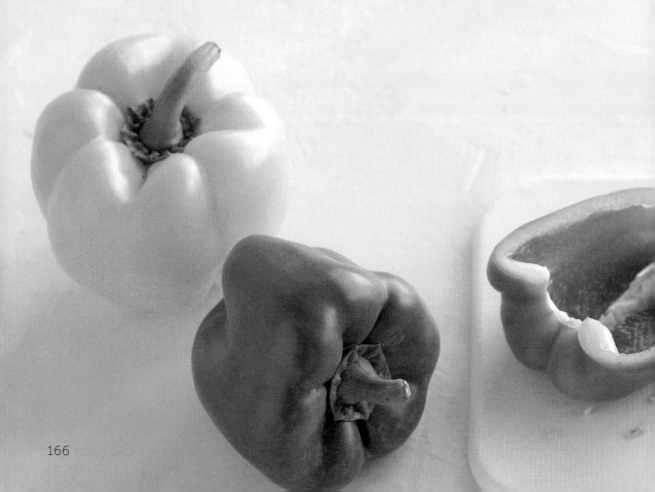

Snack ideas

Quick protein
Protein-rich foods like fish and eggs can be the simplest fast food; they are quick to cook and, combined with whole grains, ensure a good supply of the amino acids you need.

Quick snacks
Eat a small handful of mixed nuts and an apple, or snack on raw vegetables, such as cherry tomatoes, pepper strips and carrot sticks.

Nuts
Unsalted nuts and seeds are an all-round good snack. A few unsalted, unflavoured nuts help curb appetite. Containing 'good' fats, nuts (with the skin on) are high in fibre and protein and fill you up instead of sugary snacks. Be mindful that they are high in calories, but an occasional handful as a snack is a good thing. Try mixing some nuts with seeds and toasting them on a tray in a hot oven for a few minutes. Add spices such as smoked paprika, cumin or five spice for a savoury kick, and then store them in a jar.

Fruit
Strawberries can satisfy as a simple snack, or something sweet: a good choice because strawberries also contain fibre and are low calorie, packed with antioxidants and rich in vitamin C.

Other snack suggestions:
- Thinly sliced cucumber.

- Mozzarella (reduced-fat can be used, if you wish) with sliced tomato, a little drizzle of vinegar and a touch of olive oil.

- Cottage cheese with finely sliced spring or red onions; add a dash of vinegar to liven it up.

- Cabbage, carrot, shallot or onion 'slaw, using a little olive oil, mustard and vinegar (no mayo).

- Sliced boiled egg with watercress.

- Boiled eggs: these are always good in various ways, such as in salads, rice or bean mixes or just served with a simple dip like unsweetened yogurt mixed with herbs.

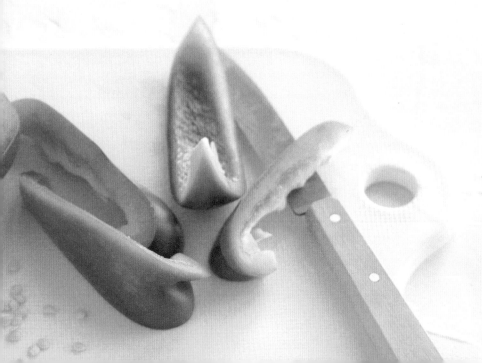

Dinner and evening options

Chicken
Chicken breast with brown rice and vegetables; this also makes a good lunch at the weekend.

Turkey
A great lean source of protein. Try the Spiced Turkey with Peppers and Tomatoes (see page 138) or the Simple Turkey & Mushroom Broth (see page 43).

Potato
Small jacket potato or sweet potato, with a small tin of reduced-sugar and -salt baked beans and salad.

Veggies
Up your veggie intake with Vegetable Scramble (see page 80), Mixed Mushroom and Chinese Noodle Soup (see page 51) or Moroccan Bean Patties (see page 99).

Fish
I like the Tandoori salmon (see page 112), Fish Tacos (see page 113) or Spiced Fish Cakes (see page 120).

Hearty stews
When it's cold outside, give these a go: Thick Bean and Dark Cabbage Stew (see page 56). Summer Vegetable Soup (see page 47) or Vegetable Tagine (see page 107).

Light meals
Dinner doesn't have to be a big meal, so try the Tomato & Feta Balls (see page 88) or Vegetable Spring Rolls (see page 86).

Dessert Options

Fruit
Fresh fruit is always a good option: blueberries, apricots, pears, apples, etc.

Ice cream
A scoop of yogurt ice cream is another way to get a sweet treat, or at home, whizz up frozen berries with frozen banana into a slushy ice. See the recipe on page 35.

Frozen
Frozen berries with frozen banana ice are a great sweet treat.

Other dessert ideas:
- Two squares of extra-bitter chocolate.

- A little unsweetened yogurt with fresh fruit.

- Frozen, pitted dates taste like a fudgy sweet.

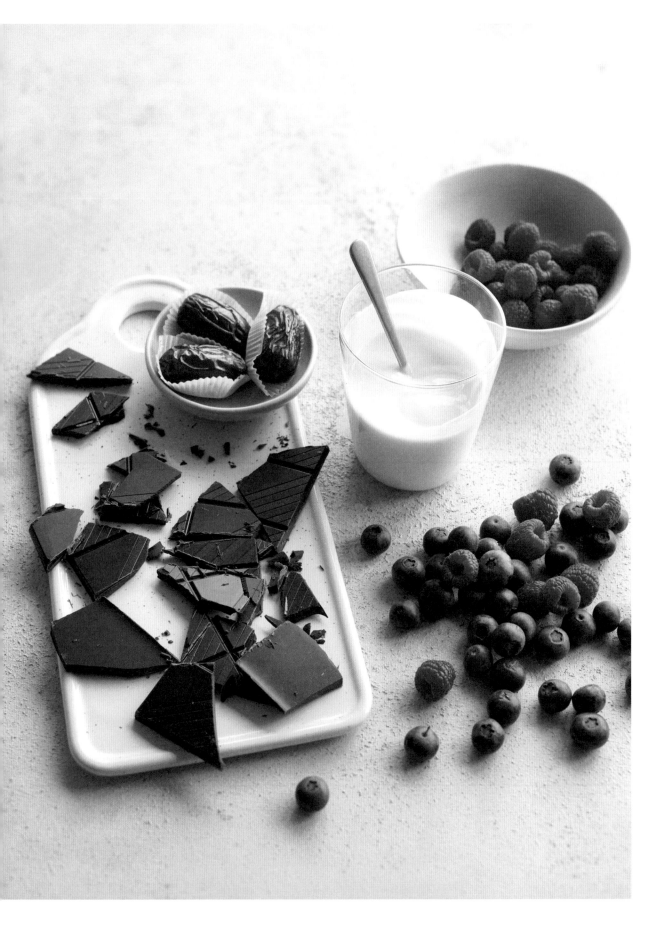

Before You Begin

In the low-calorie meal planners, each week is accompanied by a shopping list. For ease, even though only one person may be following the weight-loss plan, the list is based on serving four people. Those not trying to lose weight can add extra meals, side dishes and/or healthy snacks.

The shopping lists include fresh foods and extra items you may need to buy for the recipes that week. They do not include items such as oils, spices and tinned food that you may already have in your cupboards.

Try to shop, prepare and cook in bulk: I know this is not always possible, but it can save you a lot of time, money and stress of having to think about all your meals. It can be hard to find the time to prepare meals, and so it's a real help to cook more than you need: cooked portions can be saved or frozen to help you make less effort next time.

Already prepared ingredients can make the next meal easier and quicker to put together. I have no problem using frozen fish, meat, vegetables, rice and beans; they are very good and also good value for money. Canned foods also offer a huge variety of options, plus they are nutritious, easy to use and generally really good value for money.

Tips

Each day:
- Keep in mind a balanced plate from all the food groups.

- Target five-a-day fruit and vegetable portions.

- Keep portion sizes small, to eat less overall.

Over the week:
- Include oily fish like tandoori salmon and fish tacos.

- Add fibre from whole fruit, whole grains and plenty of green leafy veg.

Useful Store-cupboard Ingredients

Below is a handy list of store-cupboard items that you will find yourself returning to time and again as you cook the recipes in the planner and in this book.

Oils and condiments
oil – rapeseed, olive and extra
   virgin olive oil
1-calorie vegetable oil cooking
   spray
black pepper
balsamic vinegar
reduced-salt soy sauce
fish sauce
vinegar
reduced-salt stock cubes –
   chicken, fish and vegetable
tomato purée
capers
Dijon mustard
Sriracha chilli sauce
Tabasco sauce

Nuts and seeds
sunflower seeds
chia seeds
ground almonds
ground super seed mix
milled flaxseeds

Aromatics
dried oregano
dried sage
dried mixed herbs
ground allspice
ground coriander
ground cumin
ground turmeric
garam masala
dried spice mix
chilli flakes
hot smoked paprika
mild curry paste
ginger purée
black mustard seeds
black onion seeds
saffron
asafoetida
seaweed flakes
lemongrass purée
white miso paste

Cans and grains
chopped tomatoes
beans – cannellini, black beans,
   butter beans and kidney beans
lentils – green, red or brown
tuna in water
rice – Arborio, brown basmati,
   black rice, microwaveable
   sachets
rice vermicelli
pearl barley
quinoa
oats – rolled porridge and jumbo
buckwheat flakes
oat bran
wholemeal flour
gram (chickpea) flour

Baking and other useful items
granulated sweetener
honey
vanilla extract
cocoa powder
baking powder
bicarbonate of soda
espresso powder

Two Week Planner

Here are some sample low-calorie menus, using recipes from the book, to help you plan two weeks of meals. These menus are not intended for long term unless you add additional meal and snacks.

Week 1: Shopping List

Meat and fish
6 chicken breasts
2 small skinless turkey
    breast slices
4 young pheasant breasts
120g cooked or fresh prawns
900g mixed frozen seafood
500g salmon fillets

Fresh aromatics
11 yellow onions
6 red onions
4 shallots
18 spring onions
3 garlic heads (28 garlic
    cloves)
2 small fresh red chillies
5cm-piece fresh ginger
bunch of fresh mint
bunch of basil
small bunch of Thai basil
bunch of flat-leaf parsley
bunch of coriander
small bunch of fresh
    lemon thyme
small bunch of chives

Fruit and vegetables
225g sweet potato
250g waxy potatoes
1 squash
1 small swede
2 cauliflowers
400g fresh or frozen peas (or
    petits pois)
200g frozen broad beans
160g sugar snap peas or
    mangetout
5 courgettes
160g sprouting broccoli
200g beansprouts
400g medium and baby carrots
1 red or green pepper
450g mushrooms
450g button mushrooms
450g spinach
360g pak choi or Chinese leaves
700g tomatoes
1 small leek
3 celery sticks
2 Little Gem lettuce
1 ripe avocado
80g black olives
2 large limes

1 unwaxed lemon
8 small bananas
200g fresh or frozen blueberries
8 ripe plums
1 mango
watermelon slices

Eggs and dairy
18 eggs
25g mature Cheddar
15–20g Parmesan
300g unsweetened Greek-style
    yogurt
300g fat-free fromage frais
1.85 litres skimmed milk
500ml almond milk

Bread and more
wholemeal sourdough
4 sheets filo pastry

Store-cupboard extras
8 gelatine leaves
rose or orange flower water
custard powder

Day 1

Avocado & Pea Smash-up
[Page 22]

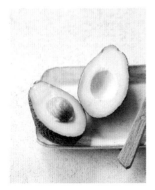

193 calories
This combo can go on toast with rocket, some sliced tomato and a splash of balsamic vinegar, plus a sprinkle of chilli flakes. Add a handful of baby spinach, or some asparagus, when in season, to boost your greens.

Vegetable Noodles with Spicy Garlic Dressing
[Page 67]

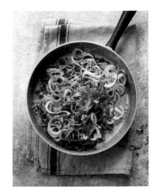

57 calories
A rainbow of courgette, carrot, sweet potato and beetroot noodles are all delicious, lower calorie and lower carb, with more fibre than noodles or pasta. Make them from scratch or buy ready-prepared.

Salmon in Miso Broth with Black Rice and Braised Greens [Page 118]

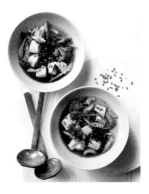

453 calories
A Japanese-inspired simple broth for a quick lunch or supper. Miso is high in salt but protein- and nutrient-rich; black rice is high in heart-healthy polyphenols and has more fibre and protein than white or brown rice.

Bitter Chocolate Muffins
[Page 152]

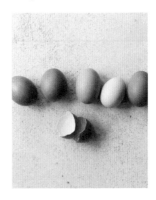

156 calories
This is a nice, simple recipe that provides a healthier snack alternative, with the majority of the fat coming from healthier sources such as eggs. Just mix the wet and dry ingredients and bake!

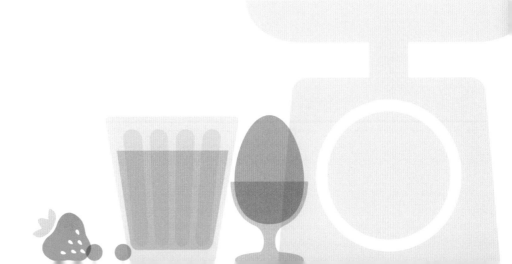

Day 2

Two Grain Porridge
[Page 31]

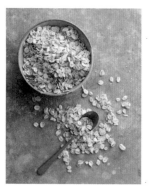

91 calories
This power porridge helps you to feel fuller, plus the fibre found in oats, beta-glucan, is linked to lowering cholesterol, and buckwheat adds a healthy variety to your diet.

Five Vegetable Curry
[Page 102]

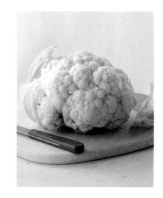

239 calories
A simple, everyday Indian curry with a combination of vegetables you can vary with the seasons. Try adding extra spices for more complex flavours.

Chicken Salad with Tomatoes, Olives and Capers [Page 65]

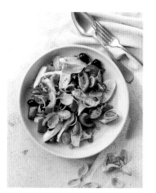

354 calories
A punchy little salad. Use the most flavoursome kind of tomatoes you can find; it will make all the difference to the taste.

Ripe mango with plain yogurt

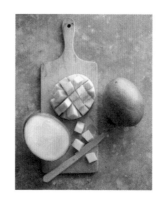

68 calories
Destone 1 mango and slice thinly. Divide between four bowls, then serve with 75g plain, unsweetened yogurt per person. The mango is naturally sweet so you don't need to add any sugar here.

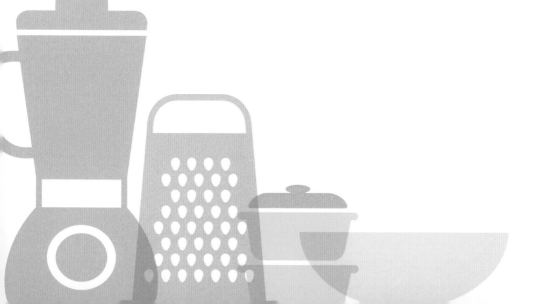

Day 3

Almond Milk Latte
[Page 38]

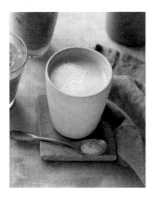

127 calories
Almond milk contains nothing more than fresh almonds and filtered water. No additives needed. The characteristics of almond milk compliment coffee well.

Potato, Herb, Tuna & Rice Frittata
[Page 117]

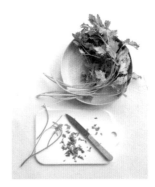

285 calories
Tuna is very versatile and very good for you. Like all canned fish, it needs little to no cooking; all you do is warm it gently so it doesn't dry out.

Fragrant Turkey Pho
[Page 132]

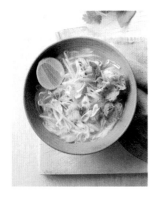

269 calories
On every street corner in Hanoi, Vietnam, they serve Pho from very early in the morning up until lunchtime. It is a very satisfying meal and is very good for you.

Plum Compote
[Page 148]

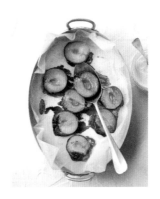

45 calories
Plums are underrated: they are packed with good nutrients; the antioxidants are concentrated in the skins, so ensure you leave these on when cooking.

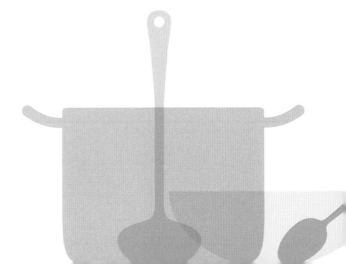

Day 4

Rock & Roller Granola
[Page 30]

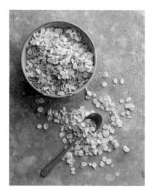

115 calories
If you don't have the time, or appetite, to sit down for breakfast in the morning, this is a liquid option for breakfast on-the-go. Try making it with the Skinny Granola recipe for extra goodness.

Minestrone Greens & Beans
[Page 44]

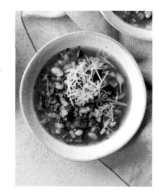

215 calories
A hearty, satisfying vegetable stew that's easy to adapt to what is in your cupboard. Feel free to switch in any beans in your cupboard: beans are lower GI than potatoes, low in fat and full of protein and fibre.

Spicy Cauliflower Rice with Prawns & Baby Spinach [Page 124]

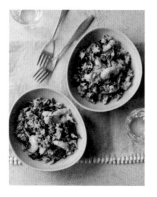

113 calories
Cauliflower is surging in popularity, from an alternative to flour in pizza dough to good old cauliflower cheese. Here it replaces rice in this veg-packed dish.

Banana Spring Rolls
[Page 158]

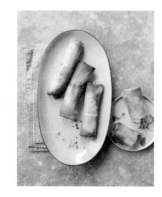

188 calories
Try freezing these in advance and cooking from frozen for an easy dessert. You get a whole banana per person here, which means there's no need to add any sugar.

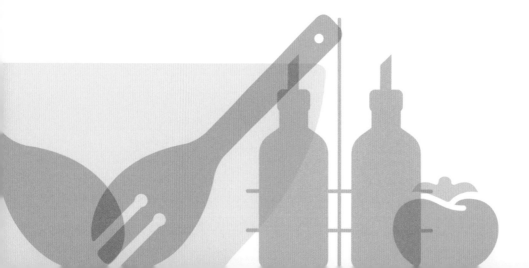

Day 5

Two Grain Porridge, served with blueberries
[Page 31]

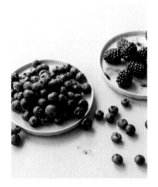

214 calories
Add 160g blueberries to this power porridge, which helps you to feel fuller, plus the fibre found in oats, beta-glucan, is linked to lowering cholesterol, and buckwheat adds a healthy variety to your diet.

Barley Soup with Allspice, Sage & Onion
[Page 55]

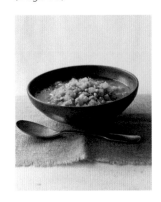

191 calories
A warming, hearty one-pot meal. Cooking in this way retains water-soluble nutrients such as B vitamins. you can also try this with kamut, spelt, freekeh or faro.

Spring Braised Chicken with Little Gem, Peas & Beans [Page 128]

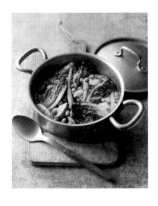

245 calories
Chicken is a rich source of carnosine, which supports the immune system. And braising lettuce not only gives a great texture but also brings a wonderful colour to the dish.

Watermelon with Saffron Yogurt, Basil & Mint [Page 154]

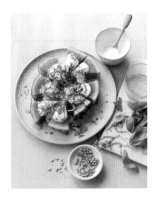

109 calories
Saffron and herbs bring a fresh, flavoursome element to this simple dessert. A great alternative to ice cream.

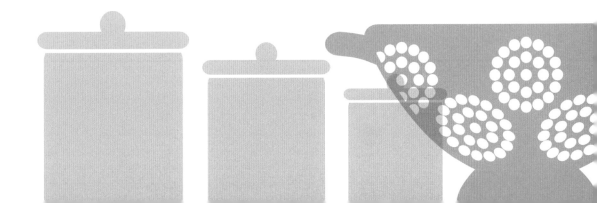

Day 6

Poached eggs on wholemeal toast

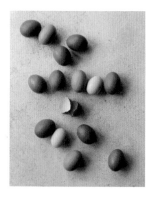

274 calories
Poach two eggs per person and serve on a slice of wholemeal toast each. Add a dash of vinegar to the water to help cook perfect poached eggs. See page 92.

Beetroot & Feta Falafels, served with pitta and salad [Page 85]

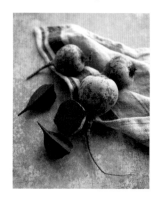

162 calories
For a light lunch: split and warm a 35g pitta bread. Stuff with one falafel, 15g chopped cucumber, rocket salad and a teaspoon of 0%-fat unsweetened Greek-style yogurt.

Really Easy Seafood & Tomato Stew
[Page 121]

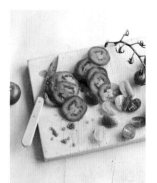

252 calories
Using frozen seafood bags is convenient, and the lycopene in tomatoes helps balance free-radicals. Plus it is easier for your body to absorb this nutrient when tomatoes are cooked.

Pannacotta
[Page 156]

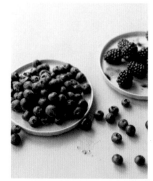

70 calories
Really easy recipe. Serve this with a few berries scattered over, or try frozen blueberries and blackcurrants, as they tend to extrude a lovely juice when defrosted.

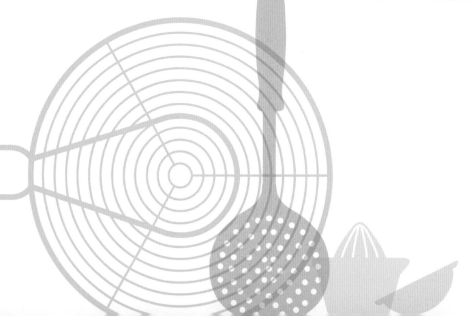

Day 7

Creamy Mushrooms on Sourdough Toast
[Page 24]

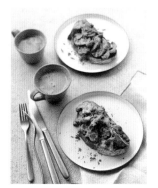

134 calories
You can use basic button mushrooms for this or mix it up with others. Mushrooms can be a source of vitamin D, which helps the body absorb calcium.

Quinoa Chinese Leaf Mushroom Bowl with Poached Eggs [Page 92]

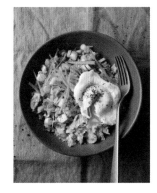

262 calories
The mix of raw and cooked ingredients in this light lunch, provide a good source of essential nutrients, and the leaves contain useful vitamins and minerals, which can help to keep blood pressure within a healthy range.

Quick Pheasant & Lentil Curry
[Page 134]

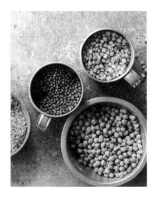

382 calories
This easy and very quick curry only takes a few minutes to cook. The lentils are filling thanks to their high fibre content, so a smaller portion size goes a long way.

Vanilla Blancmange
[Page 157]

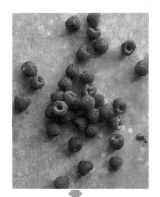

139 calories
A sugar-free version of blancmange: I have to say, it works really well if you fancy a light dessert and serve with a little fresh fruit.

Week 2: Shopping List

Meat and fish
200g chicken breast
4 chicken or other lean
 meat burgers
4 low-fat chicken sausages
450g squid
300g turkey breast

Fresh aromatics
12 yellow onions
3 red onions
3 shallots
10 spring onions
2 garlic heads (18 cloves)
1 red chilli
6cm-piece fresh ginger
4 bunches of basil
2 bunches of chives
2 bunches of coriander
2 bunches of parsley
bunch of tarragon
small bunch of Thai basil

Fruit and vegetables
2 small potatoes
9 sweet potatoes
1 celeriac
1 small cauliflower
3 aubergines

7 courgettes
5 carrots
½ small red cabbage
150g frozen peas
200g green beans
200g mangetout
peppers – 1 orange, 1 green,
 4 red and 2 yellow
75g red chicory
220g baby spinach
150g lettuce
½ avocado
4 celery sticks
125g cucumber
1 small fennel bulb
tomatoes – 5 medium and
 160g cherry
2 lemons
2 limes
10 bananas
250g blueberries or blackberries
400g strawberries
320g frozen dark cherries
320g frozen mixed berries

Eggs and dairy
10 eggs
50g Parmesan
30g reduced-fat Cheddar

325g 0%-fat unsweetened
 Greek-style yogurt
2 tablespoons low-fat crème
 fraîche
8 tablespoons cottage cheese
400g low-fat unsweetened live
 yogurt or kefir
700ml skimmed milk
500ml almond milk

Bread
2 slices seeded wholegrain
 bread
4 wholemeal buns
4 sheets filo pastry

Store-cupboard extras
100g granola, ideally homemade
15g dried sliced mushrooms
50g crunchy peanut butter
10g dark chocolate
125ml sparkling water

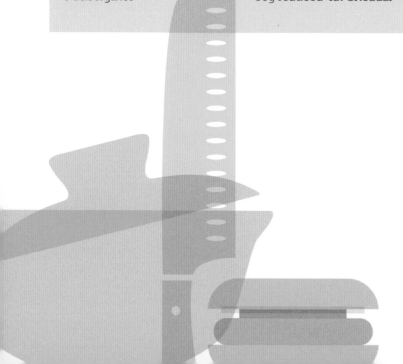

Day 8

Egg Salad on Toast
[Page 28]

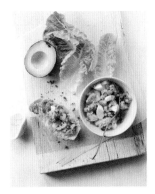

175 calories
Instead of mayo, mashed avocado is used for this creamy, light breakfast. Spread on wholemeal bread and enjoy!

Summer Vegetable Soup
[Page 47]

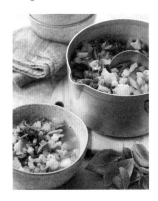

155 calories
A veg-packed summer soup, with ginger, lemongrass and oregano. There should be so much veg that the spoon stands up in the pot.

Blueprint Burgers, served with
Sweet Potato Fries [Pages 140 & 71]

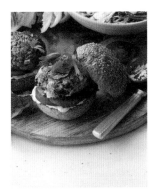

542 calories
Keep your burgers on the healthy side with a wholemeal bun, griddled chicken breasts and lots of veg layers. Sweet potatoes have significantly more potassium, calcium and vitamin K than normal potatoes.

Dairy Berry Power Smoothie
[Page 35]

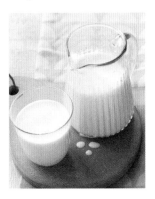

132 calories
Use frozen fruit for a thick and refreshingly ice cold smoothie: you'll probably need to eat it with a spoon!

Day 9

Two Grain Porridge, served with blueberries
[Page 31]

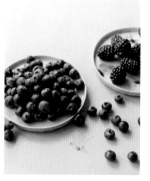

214 calories
Add 160g blueberries to this power porridge, which helps you to feel fuller, plus the fibre found in oats, beta-glucan, is linked to lowering cholesterol, and buckwheat adds a healthy variety to your diet.

Herb Broth with Spring Onions & Ginger
[Page 42]

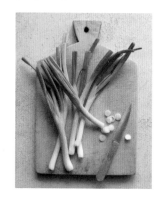

67 calories
A simple soup that you can make and leave in the fridge until needed. This recipe is packed with nutritious vegetables and the flavour mostly comes from the herbs and ginger.

Twice Baked Sweet Potatoes with Sausages & Beans [Page 136]

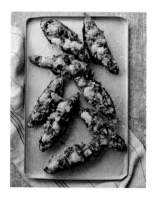

358 calories
Twice-baked jackets turn a simple baked potato into a full main course. Microwave for 4–5 minutes first, to cut the cooking time in half.

Strawberries on Sweet Cottage Cheese
[Page 153]

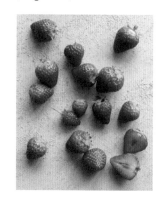

93 calories
This is incredibly simple for a snack or something sweet, and provides nutritious protein, fibre and vitamins. Strawberries are also low calorie, packed with antioxidants and rich in vitamin C.

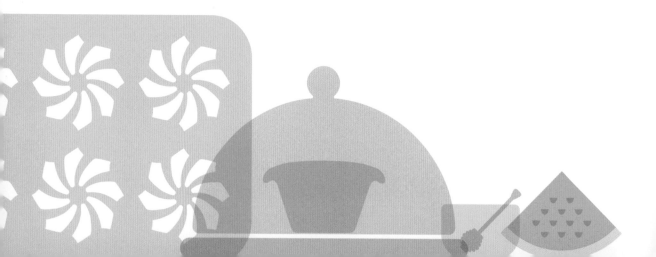

Day 10

Almond Milk Latte
[Page 38]

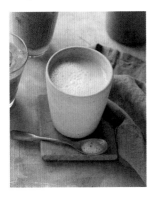

127 calories
Great for a morning coffee break, or chill it down for an iced summer drink. Try adding spices or infusing with a chai tea bag for a different flavour.

Fennel Slaw Salad, served on wholemeal toast [Page 68]

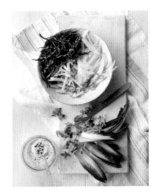

144 calories
Add a slice of wholemeal toast to this side salad to make it a light lunch. This colourful salad came from the idea of tweaking coleslaw to be a bit healthier.

Celeriac Risotto
[Page 108]

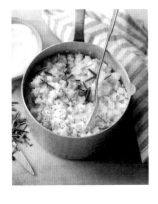

225 calories
This recipe shows you can produce a great, hearty main course with no meat or fish protein at all: praise the veg!

Chocolate Power Balls
[Page 147]

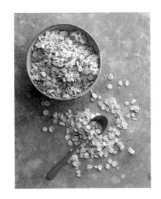

100 calories
Have one of these for when you fancy something sweet and only chocolate will hit the spot. The dates offer a natural source of sugar and fibre, instead of commercially made sweets.

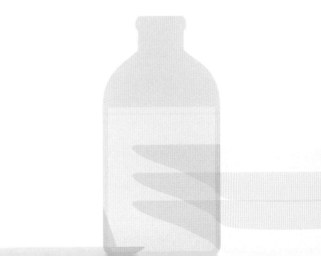

Day 11

Roasted Red Pepper & Sardines on Toast
[Page 27]

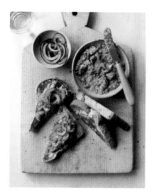

196 calories
Canned sardines are inexpensive; they are a great source of calcium, as well as protein, and a top up for your diet of omega-3 from the oily fish. Keep a batch of roasted peppers in the freezer for other recipes, like this one.

Easy Spiced Turkey with Peppers & Tomatoes
[Page 138]

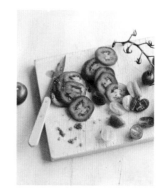

164 calories
Just simmer all the vegetables and spices, then sauté the turkey and add that's it. No browning: just pop it all in and get on with your life...

Aubergine & Bean Burgers, served with Mexican Refried Black Beans [Pages 91 & 104]

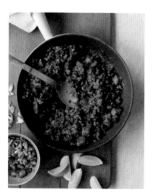

214 calories
To avoid aubergines absorbing lots of oil when cooking, pre-cook them slightly in the microwave first. Tomatoes are used instead of lard to make the Mexican refried black beans a bit healthier.

Fruity Ice Cream Power Smoothie
[Page 35]

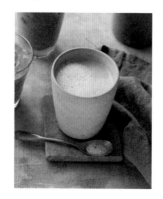

68 calories
This is more of a cheat's ice cream and makes a great pudding. Banana is a magic ingredient for sweetening and thickening that can be conveniently kept in the freezer ready to use from frozen.

Day 12

Oat & Chia Breakfast Pots
[Page 32]

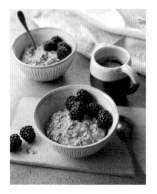

221 calories
Chia seeds are an excellent source of plant proteins and fibre, and make for a great variation on the popular overnight oats: make the night before and these are ready to eat in the morning.

Vegetable Noodles with Spicy Garlic Dressing
[Page 67]

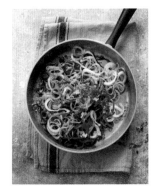

57 calories
A rainbow of courgette, carrot, sweet potato and beetroot noodles are all delicious, lower calorie and lower carb, with more fibre than noodles or pasta. Make them from scratch or buy ready-prepared.

Sautéed Squid with Yogurt & Lime
[Page 123]

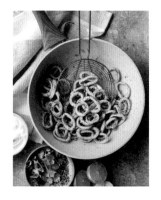

111 calories
Cook this dish in batches to keep the heat in the pan and give the squid a nice colour. Frozen squid is fine and actually makes for more tender squid.

Silky Chocolate Mousse
[Page 151]

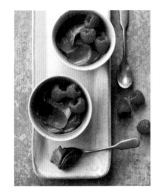

75 calories
Using silken tofu to create a creamy texture means that this dessert is vegan and low calorie but still tastes like a chocolatey treat.

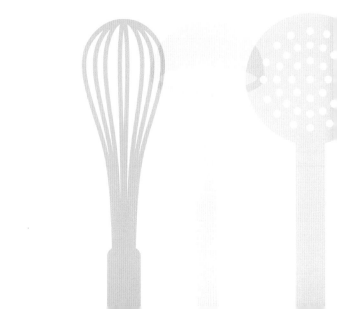

Day 13

Baked Green Eggy Pots
[Page 23]

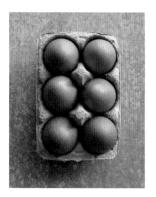

101 calories
These are baked to reduce the added fat in cooking. They're also packed with protein, which is great for keeping you satisfied and less likely to reach for a snack before lunch.

Tortilla Muffins
[Page 83]

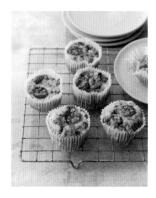

73 calories
Great for using up leftover bits of cooked veg. The egg adds a nutritious boost of protein.

Braised Aubergines with Spiced Butterbeans & Crispy Garlic [Page 96]

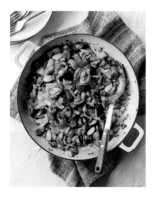

123 calories
This recipe starts the cooking process with water to cut out 90 per cent of the oil that you would normally use, which can be sucked up when cooking aubergine.

Banana, Oat & Peanut Cookie Balls
[Page 146]

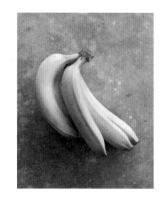

145 calories
Three simple ingredients make a soft, cookie-style portion, for when you want something to nibble instead of a premade snack, which can contain less healthy sources of fat and sugar.

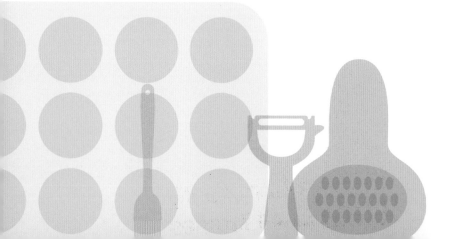

Day 14

Savoury Socca Pancakes
[Page 89]

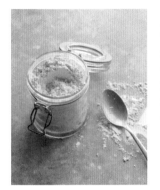

156 calories
This savoury pancake is similar to a flatbread originating in Nice, France. Using chickpea flour means this is both gluten-free and vegan.

Chicken Meatballs with Garlic, Herbs & Paprika, served with asparagus [Page 131]

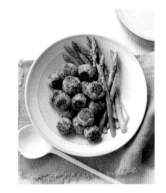

215 calories
Though these meatballs are fried, they are low in fat. Serve with 100g steamed asparagus each.

Mixed Bean Chilli
[Page 103]

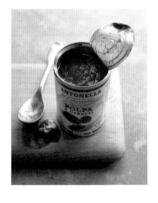

239 calories
Tweak as you please here: there are so many versions that pretty much anything goes. Just pack it with veg and you're good.

Banana Spring Rolls
[Page 158]

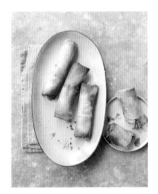

188 calories
Try freezing these in advance and cooking from frozen for an easy dessert. You get a whole banana per person here, which means there's no need to add any sugar.

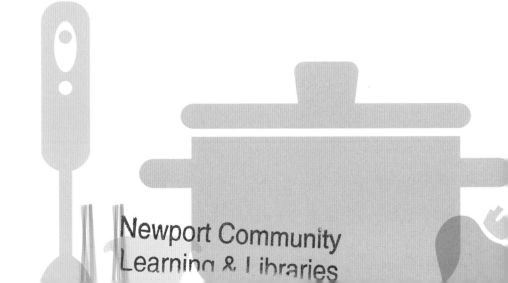

Index

DIABETES MEAL PLANNER

Acknowledgements

Any book is a huge amount of work to put together and I certainly couldn't do it on my own. Bea Harling is the best in the business by far and I increasingly rely on her help, opinion and knowledge to get this book over the line. Judith Hannam oversees the whole shebang and keeps me well and truly in line, whilst letting me get on with it, thank you. Luigi Bonomi and John Rush for sorting all the nitty gritty and being great friends. The fabulous KB team: Kate Whitaker (photographer), Annie Rigg (food stylist), Paul Palmer-Edwards (designer), Claire Rogers (project editor), Florence Filose (editorial assistant) and Lou Blair (nutritional analysis). Finally, a big thank you to DUK, Shirley Quinn and Emma Elvin.

PiLL 17-09-2020.